Contents

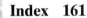
Appendices

Glossary   157

Index   161

Acknowledgments

Thanks to my "boss" and friend Jan Dinkel, Dean, Shasta College for her appreciation and support of my trials and tribulations. Thank you to my students for their participation and contributions. I also want to thank John for his intelligent humor, my sons Kris, Lenny, Rik, and as always my mom Joanne.

Vickie J. Kimbrough RDH, MBA

I would like to thank my co-author and colleague, Vickie Kimbrough. Thank you for your guiding hand and partnership through this project. Also Jan Dinkel, Dean, Shasta College—your high expectations and standards have helped me to expect more of myself, as well. And especially my husband, Brett, thank you for your constant support and encouragement—your belief in me keeps me focused.

Karen Henderson RDH, BA

Reviewers

Julie Bencosme, RDH, MA, CHES
Assistant Professor
Dental Hygiene
Hostos Community College
Bronx, New York

Judith A. Crooks-Cheney, RDH, BA
Department of Dental Hygiene
Fresno City College
Fresno, California

Deborah Durham, RDH, MPA
Chairperson
Department of Dental Hygiene
Temple College
Temple, Texas

Donna Eastabrooks, RDH, M.Ed.
Associate Professor
Dental Hygiene Program
Manor College
Jenkintown, Pennsylvania

Suzanne M. Edenfield, RDH, Ed.D.
Associate Professor
Department of Dental Hygiene
Armstrong Atlantic State University
Savannah, Georgia

Lynette M. Engeswick, RDH, MS
Chairperson
Department of Dental Hygiene
Minnesota State University Mankato
Mankato, Minnesota

Chris French Beatty, RDH, Ph.D.
Associate Professor
Department of Dental Hygiene
Texas Woman s University
Denton, Texas

Judith A. Hall, RDH, BS
Chairperson
Department of Dental Hygiene
Delaware Technical and Community
  College
Wilmington, Delaware

Debby Kurtz-Weidinger, RDH, M.Ed.
Faculty
Department of Dental Programs
Phoenix College
Phoenix, Arizona

Kristin L. Mallory, RDH, M.Ed.
Assistant Professor and Chairperson
Department of Dental Hygiene
West Virginia University Institute
  of Technology
Montgomery, West Virginia

Angelina E. Riccelli, RDH, MS
Associate Professor
School of Dental Medicine
University of Pittsburgh
Pittsburgh, Pennsylvania

Barbara M. Sidel, RDH, MA
Instructor
Dental Hygiene Department
Delaware Technical and Community
  College
Dover, Delaware

Rebecca Stolberg, RDH, MS
Department Chair and Assistant Professor
Department of Dental Hygiene
Eastern Washington University
Spokane, Washington

Introduction

One of the most challenging tasks for oral health care providers is educating and motivating those they are caring for. Although numerous changes have occurred in dentistry in regard to technology and creating an environment that helps to alleviate apprehension, the key to making all patients partners in their oral health remains illusive.

The purpose of this text is to provide oral health practitioners and students a better understanding of current dental health in consumers, lifestyle influences on systemic health, trends in health perceptions from infancy to older adulthood, and how to bridge the gap in communication styles to better work with patients, community organizations, and other health care colleagues. By doing so, all aspects of health can be used to improve the systemic and oral health in people of all ages and demographics.

During health education, be it in dental hygiene, dentistry, nursing, childhood education, or geriatric care, there are many ways to approach patient motivation so that individuals take ownership of their overall health. Many practitioners have found that a number of their patients remain unmotivated and the reasons are diverse. What does it take, not only to get the message across, but also to have the patients incorporate a new value for their overall health? Many educational programs provide case studies that will assist students in developing the communication skills necessary to work with a diverse spectrum of people. In addition, students are provided with statistics that can aid in broadening their oral health presentations to consumers seen during their dental hygiene education. Community health courses are designed to give students the opportunity to reach people of all ages within their respective communities and present important oral health information. So how can all who enter healthcare fields use these tools in an ongoing basis?

It is the authors' hope that new graduates as well as current practitioners find new approaches to health care education from the information provided in this text. Health among the young and old is deteriorating. All health care providers must send the same message: Oral health is linked to systemic health. As new graduates from the dental and medical fields enter the workforce, it will be of utmost importance to incorporate this message within them so that those they treat throughout their career have the information and tools necessary to become a partner in their own well-being—for life.

NOTE: The authors recognize and acknowledge that many educational programs use the terms "patient" and "client" both interchangeably and individually. The authors have elected to use the term "patient" throughout the text to maintain smooth reading transition. It is not meant to imply that all those given dental hygiene services and education have a condition or disease.

1

Current Trends in Dental Health

Objectives

Upon reading the material in this chapter, you will be able to

1. Incorporate systemic health links into patient education of oral health.
2. Discuss barriers to traditional oral health care delivery.
3. Identify federal programs addressing health care.
4. Recognize and discuss the significance of the Surgeon General's Report on Oral Health.
5. Discuss effective methods to include the medical professional in recognizing oral health links to systemic health.

Introduction

The following information is designed to give sufficient demographic information so that individuals designing and providing oral health education to patients have the opportunity to effectively substantiate the importance of excellent oral health. Many factors learned in community dental health courses during dental hygiene education become the foundation for oral health education to patients. Enhancing and augmenting such material allows students to become adept in the background information needed to ensure patients significant reasons for improving their oral health status through compliance. For many years consumers have viewed the dental hygienist as the "person who does the cleaning." The majority of consumers are unaware of the extensive education their dental hygienist has obtained. When discussing oral health, the educator, whether a student or a seasoned practitioner, will want to stay current on health statistics and trends as it affects oral health.

Dental Health and Systemic Health

In the late 1990s, the dental and medical communities were hit with a revolutionary research outcome that showed a link between oral health and systemic health. The culprit: bacteria. Today, it all seems second nature. Many say that the eyes are the windows to the soul, which means that the mouth could be seen as the window to the body—or better yet, the door. It only makes sense that what a person ingests will lead to either a healthy lifestyle or an unhealthy lifestyle. The oral cavity is not separated from the rest of the body and why it took centuries to realize that oral bacteria could contribute to declining health may be forever a mystery. There will be short-term and long-term effects of what one does today as a result of their diet and exercise routine. Yet many people would rather live for today than worry about tomorrow. For the dental professional it will be imperative to influence patients to make a change in their eating habits if they want to save their teeth. For other health care providers it will be imperative to influence patients to make a change in their lifestyle in order to live a longer, healthier life.

What is **oral health**? Is it the same for everyone since many people have different oral conditions, such as missing teeth, restored teeth, and so on? These are good questions to consider, since everyone has different existing conditions. According to the World Health Organization (1982), "Oral health is a standard of the oral and related tissues which enables an individual to eat, speak and socialize without active disease, discomfort or embarrassment and which contributes to general well-being." Society in general has always viewed a pretty smile as an indicator for good teeth and healthy gums. Yet statistics are indicating otherwise and all professional dental organizations have begun to advocate for optimal oral health. Few people die from oral diseases, yet the cost of treating it is astronomical at all levels: individuals, families, third-party insurance companies, and government agencies. For example, in the United Kingdom, costs for treating dental disease outweigh the cost for treating all cancers and heart disease (East Sussex, Brighton and Hove Health Authority, 2000). The American Academy of General Dentistry is among those to promote the importance of oral health, recognizing that more than 90 percent of all systemic diseases have oral manifestations and that oral infections can affect major organs (bacterial endocarditis). The Surgeon General reported that some type of periodontal disease or gingivitis affects more than 75 percent of the population. The statistics reveal the significance of the dental professional in preventing and treating oral diseases, as they may be the first health care provider to diagnose a problem. The importance for regular oral health care and education becomes imperative for improving oral health and will impact the well-being of all.

Since the late 1990s, as previously mentioned, it has become more apparent with continued research that not only is cardiovascular disease linked to oral disease, so is respiratory disease and preterm low birth weight (PLBW) babies. There are good or normal bacteria thriving in the same environment as infectious microorganisms. As medical research continues to assist in better understanding this link, oral health practitioners must continue to educate patients in the relationship that exists between oral and systemic health. Of course, bacteria are not the single influence to systemic diseases that take the life of millions each year. Other known risk factors still include stress, tobacco use, high blood pressure, family history, genetics, weight, alcohol use, and lack of physical activity. There are more and more risk factors being discovered each year that can shorten one's lifespan.

LINK 1

Cardiovascular disease may be exacerbated by periodontal inflammation. The National Institute of Dental Craniofacial Research (NIDCR) reports that scientific theories site opportunistic infectious bacteria that colonizes in the mouth form **biofilms.** These biofilms can activate white blood cells releasing inflammatory mediators that may contribute to heart disease and stroke. Diseased periodontium serves as a reservoir for inflammatory mediators that can enter the circulation and either enhance or perpetuate systemic effects (Lamster & Lalla, 2004, p. 11). This inflammation, along with other risk factors, taxes the body's ability to fight systemic disease. In a periodontal pocket, bacterial biofilm directly contacts ulcerated epithelium (p. 11). The more advanced the periodontal condition, the more surface area for bacteria to enter the bloodstream. According to the American Academy of Periodontology (AAP, 2003), more recent studies are now indicating that elevated levels of C-reactive proteins are better at determining the risk for cardiovascular disease associated with periodontal disease. The liver makes c-reactive proteins after being triggered by the number of bacterial by-products in the bloodstream. This trigger response system causes increased arterial inflammation.

LINK 2

In health care education programs students learn how to identify symptoms of systemic diseases. For example, diabetes is rising in young adults and children by what appears to be poor diet and lack of exercise (see Chapter 2). Diabetes can go undetected for several years. Destructive inflammatory processes that occur with periodontal diseases are more closely intertwined for individuals with poor or uncontrolled diabetes. Periodontal disease is likely to develop as a result of depressed immune systems, which then can initiate a cycle of overall poor systemic health. Over the past two decades, there has been more evidence indicating diabetes as a precursor to periodontal disease. In 1993, periodontitis was proposed as the sixth complication of diabetes (Lamster, 2004, p. 12) Controlling oral bacteria associated with inflammation that contributes to systemic bacteria will be important in overall health just as the need to control diabetes. If a graphic could be created for patients to visualize the chain of events, it may look something like Figure 1.1.

LINK 3

Preterm low birth weight (PLBW) in babies is directly related to infant mortality and other health problems (Perry, Beemsterboer, & Taggart, 2001). The first indication of this link was identified in 1996 by Offenbacher and colleagues, and subsequent studies have resulted in similar findings (Lamster & Lalla, 2004, p. 12). In pregnant women, some studies have shown that PLBW is a result of women having active periodontitis and the fact that the mother's body will secrete anti-inflammatory agents such as **prostaglandins** in response to an infection. It is theorized that these oral pathogens release toxins that reach the placenta via the mother's circulatory system and interfere with fetal growth and development (http://www.nidr.nih.gov). Women with periodontal disease showed up to an eight-fold greater chance of having PLBW infants than a mother without periodontal disease

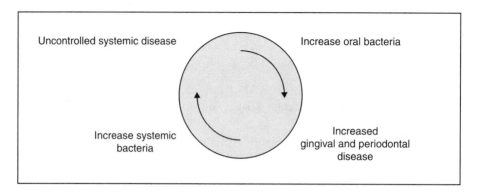

Uncontrolled systemic disease

Increase oral bacteria

Increase systemic
bacteria

Increased
gingival and periodontal
disease

FIGURE 1.1 How oral and systemic health and bacteria influence each other.

(Brooke, 2003). The NIDCR has supported researchers' estimates that as many as 18 percent of 250,000 premature low birth weight infants born in the United States each year may be attributed to infectious oral disease. This indicates a need to educate expectant mothers. By doing so, the mother-to-be will have the information needed to maintain optimal oral hygiene during the stages of her gestation so that the baby is born at a healthy weight.

LINK 4

Respiratory illnesses are more prevalent in older populations, especially those in long-term care facilities, nursing homes, and assisted living environments. For example, studies done in Europe and the United States in the mid-1990s indicated that as many as 10 percent of 65- to 69-year-olds are functionally dependent and that percentage rises with age (Henry et al., 1995). It is an unfortunate fact that the oral health status of institutionalized elderly persons is markedly poorer than those who may remain independent and reside with family or their community. The prevalence of caries, periodontitis, and edentulism is a serious concern as it only exacerbates the amount of oral microorganisms that will affect any systemic conditions already existing in these patients. It is common for many elderly individuals to acquire pneumonia and other upper respiratory illnesses while residing in a long-term care facility. When oral bacteria increase, so does the chance of pneumonia and chronic obstructive pulmonary diseases (COPD). These can be life-threatening issues, especially in those who are immunocompromised. Adequate oral health care, including dental restorations and prosthetic appliances, will be imperative for older adults to maintain the highest quality of life for as long as possible.

The U.S. Surgeon General's Report: Oral Health in America, released in May 2000, was a huge breakthrough with the information and statistics needed to support what many health care providers were documenting for years. Among the vast information presented on disparities and access to health care delivery (see Chapter 2), for the first time ever oral and systemic health were linked in their importance to the general well-being of the American public. The Surgeon General points out that oral disease has become a "silent epidemic" among the nation's most vulnerable: poor children, older adults, and racial and ethnic minority groups (U.S. Dept. of Health and Human Services, 2000, p. 1). As science links oral disease to systemic diseases, it becomes imperative for all health care providers to incorporate current information into their patient treatment plan and education. Health care providers are only one part in improving the nation's overall health status. Consumers must understand that they are the ones who hold the key to a healthy lifestyle and lifespan. This applies to every child, adult, and elderly individual. Oral diseases do not discriminate. It is broad spectrum, just as bacteria is broad spectrum. Until consumers have easier access to the dental care and education needed, disease will continue to have the upper hand.

The definition of "health" as documented by the World Health Organization in 1948 states, "a complete state of physical, mental, and social well-being, and not just the absence of infirmity." In order to accomplish a state of health, oral health must parallel. One cannot be obtained without the other as they are meshed in all aspects and levels of disease and health processes. So what does all this mean to the new graduate and the licensed practitioner? With Internet resources readily at hand (see Appendix D) and numerous published articles on oral and systemic health, current scientific information and statistics can be found to provide the background needed to reach the individual or specialty group so that the link between systemic and oral health education is understood and accepted by the average consumer. Communities are in need of licensed health care workers that will take the time to educate those who are battling systemic diseases and have the need to improve their oral health and vice versa. Dental professionals continuously educate and treat all levels of oral disease, yet may be limited in their knowledge of systemic diseases. Medical professionals have a diverse background in systemic conditions and may be limited in their oral health knowledge. By coming together, both medical and dental professionals can provide broad-based health education that will improve overall consumer health in their respective communities

So how can the dental hygiene student begin to use all this information when designing patient education, or education for specific target groups? It will be essential to have a good understanding of oral disease etiology, risk behaviors (discussed in Chapter 9), and identified systemic conditions in order to address the current oral health status of individuals, and the modifications necessary to gain improvement.

Oral Health and the Dental Hygiene Process of Care

As previously stated, students learn that the dental hygiene diagnosis is significant as it provides a process that assists in determining the etiology of current oral conditions and risk behaviors for periodontal disease and caries, and allows the clinician to gather sufficient data or perform a risk assessment that can identify unmet oral education and needs of the patient. The dental hygienist can then design the appropriate treatment plan and home care therapy for each individual. Being able to identify risk behaviors will allow the dental professional to help the patient recognize them and play a significant role in eliminating them. For the dental hygienist this task is huge, as educating and motivating each patient requires a long-term partnership. When patients realize how important it is to become an active participant in their own oral health, they will contribute to improving their overall health.

Many dental health practitioners observe what appears to be a gap between the dental and medical professionals regarding consumer education of oral and systemic health links. As each dental visit requires the practitioner to review and or update the medical history, there may be indications that warrant a referral to their medical professional. Partnering with the medical profession may assist the dental practitioner to provide optimal care and planning for each patient. For those in the medical field, partnering with dental professionals can also broaden the scope of health care delivery. A suggestion can be made from the dental health care provider to the medical provider to incorporate small but significant changes into a medical visit. For example, each time a patient visits the medical office, the nurse or nursing assistant employs the practice of taking blood pressure, and may also ask routine questions that the physician will review prior to meeting with that patient. If the nurse or assistant incorporates questions regarding their dental history (see Figure 1.2), the patient can be appropriately referred to a dental professional when and if necessary. This cooperative approach to health care is trend-setting and provides the best approach to health care delivery as a whole. Many pediatricians make it a practice to view the oral cavity of babies and toddlers during well-baby visits. This is done to check the eruption of deciduous teeth and to make sure the baby's oral condition is normal. These visits with mother and baby are an excellent opportunity for the physician to refer them to a pedodontist or family dentist initiating the start of regular oral health visits.

An important fact to keep in mind during one's dental hygiene education is that very few consumers have been exposed to information linking oral and systemic health or disease. Although health professionals have known this for several years, the average consumer, at best, may have been exposed by brief press releases via newspaper articles or television news reports. Additionally, the majority of Americans do not seek regular dental care due to numerous factors to be discussed later in this chapter. More often the consumer benefits when oral health care providers as well as those in the medical field incorporate questions relating to the oral–systemic health link during dental treatment and annual medical examinations.

Do you have sensitive teeth?
Do you have bleeding gums? When were they last examined?
Do you have oral piercing?
How often are you brushing per day?
Do you see a dentist or a dental hygienist on a regular basis?
When was your last oral examination?
When was your last dental cleaning?

FIGURE 1.2 Questions the Medical Professional can Include to Help Determine the Need for Dental Attention.

Health care practitioners want to be successful in improving overall health. Therefore, patients must understand that they have the most important role: compliance. During clinical training in school, many students meet patients that do not know the name or dose of their medication. Consumers tend to rely on the expertise of the health care provider. The savvy patient will ask pertinent questions to ensure a thorough understanding of treatment. Yet practitioners still observe the consumer not understanding or refusing to be responsible for their health care. When both students and practitioners take the time to educate consumers on aspects of oral and systemic health, they can realize the role in their own health, making those in the dental and medical fields excellent resources for information.

For the dental professional a thorough understanding of the dental hygiene process of care is essential. It is the opportunity to collect significant information for understanding the oral health history of each patient that will determine both the etiology of current oral conditions as well as designing a treatment plan and patient education needs. It is the opportunity to partner with each patient for improving oral health, which in turn influences improvement of overall systemic health and well-being.

An Overview of Barriers to Improved Oral Health

Many health education institutions such as dental, medical, dental hygiene, nursing schools, and others who have the opportunity to house their own clinic or hospital for teaching purposes generally open their doors to the public. This serves two purposes: teaching and learning opportunities for enrolled students and access to health care delivery for the consumer. Healthcare is costly. Thus when teaching institutions are able to extend student-performed services to the public, the consumer not only contributes to student learning they are also able to take advantage of quality health care at discounted fees. As a participant they are likely getting some of the best health care available, as teaching institutions are excellent resources for dental and medical research and/or information.

Even though teaching institutions do what they can there are not enough of them to handle the 43 million Americans without health benefits. There are a multitude of factors that prevent consumers from seeking health care services regardless of health care coverage. According to the Surgeon General's Report, reasons included fear, cost, access problems, have no teeth, felt that the health visit was not important, lack of insurance coverage, and income status (pp. 83–86). And 46.8 percent of those reporting for the study stated that they had no perceived dental problem, thus did not see the need to visit their dental health professional. Preventive oral health care continues to hold little value for the majority of consumers. Access to care is a major factor for those who are not covered by dental insurance, on state or federal assistance programs, and families in the low-income bracket or living at or below the poverty line. It is also a major challenge to dental organizations. What does access to care mean? It means that there are not enough facilities or providers willing to take on providing health or dental care for consumers who do not have health coverage, are low-income, or on federal/state assistance.

Economic Barriers

Consumers facing economic challenges are unable to seek dental care until it becomes absolutely necessary, which may be in the form of a dental emergency. More often to these individuals, maintaining the costs of their home and feeding their family is more important, and rightly so. The percentage of persons in all age brackets reporting cost as a factor in seeking oral health care was 13.7, 19.1% of which was attributed to those ranging from 18 to 34 years of age. As one might surmise, this age bracket represents many who are no longer covered by their parents' insurance upon leaving home or graduating from college, and may not have employment benefits that include health care. The cost to employers to provide health and dental benefits can be prohibitive to the employer, especially those deemed small businesses. Statistics gathered by the Center for Disease Control and released in the National Employer Health Survey indicated that as of 1993, 52 percent of private-sector establishments sponsored group health insurance and 58 percent of employees participated in their health plans. Additionally, the report goes on to identify that of the 4.5 million self-employed individuals, 31 percent were uninsured (http://www.cdc.gov). (As of the writing of this text, this was the most current information.) The cost for health benefits to the employee in order to participate in a plan offered by their employers averages about $1,200 annually. This is only the cost of premium payments. The employer must also contribute what is typically an equal amount for each employee. Therefore, oftentimes when economic fluctuations occur in the nation, both the employer and employee could suffer the repercussions, which typically ranges from increased fees to elimination of health benefits.

As of September 2003, the U.S. Census Bureau reported a poverty rate of 12.1 percent for 2002. The Bureau also reported that the poverty rate and the number of poor increased among several population groups: married couples, Caucasians, people between 18 to 64 years of age, and Native American families. This resulted in an increase of 1.7 million people for a final count of 34.6 million categorized as poor in 2002 (U.S. Census Bureau, 2003). When families are in financial stress, preventive oral health care finds a lower position on the priority list. Those who obtain dental care will be those who are in pain or who have a dental emergency. And statistics indicate that the majority of low-income families live with untreated decay, the majority being children.

Access/Workforce Barriers

There are other disparities in oral health care as well. Many professionals living in rural areas prefer to work more closely to home versus commuting to outlying areas that may be sparsely populated. In some areas across the nation, there may be a maldistribution of dental providers and perhaps even a true shortage. Facilities that offer dental care for economically challenged families are few and far between in cities all across America. The reasons are two-fold: dental professionals cannot get reimbursed at an adequate level to meet the cost of operations, and states are unable to build and finance such facilities due to limited funds in their budgets. Many states cannot meet the health care needs of their consumers on financial assistance programs. This dilemma only increases the number of children and adults who cannot access dental/medical care. The gap between providers and facilities to the number of consumers needing services continues to widen and the long-term prognosis to alleviating this gap is poor.

Age Barriers

Then there is the elderly population. With the lifespan of Americans increasing, more individuals will find themselves on a fixed income upon retirement. Depending on the amount of monthly income for these individuals, rising numbers of elderly are unable to seek dental care. If placed in a long-term care facility, the quality of oral health declines as a result of decreased dental care. As previously discussed, the presence of caries and poor periodontal conditions lead to more patients in need of dental care. Adding to this problem is the reluctance of caregivers to provide proper oral health care on a daily basis. Consideration must also be given to transportation issues, patient conditions, lack of dental health plans, and lack of dental professionals willing or able to provide dental care in the facility itself.

Cultural Barriers

Barriers to dental care also come in the form of cultural and family values. These values play a role in how consumers will seek dental care over their lifetime. The diversity of ethnic cultures in America is represented in highly populated areas and presents a challenge for licensed practitioners to learn and understand how each culture views oral and systemic health. It will be important for the dental professional to inquire about existing oral health practices to grasp an idea of the values held within any particular culture or family. For example, many ethnic cultures exist in extended family units where the grandparents are residing with children and grandchildren. Thus values and ideals are passed down within that unit and continue in subsequent family units. Preventive care may not be held in high regard within certain cultures or family values. Additionally, the values of a child's parents will be key to the values of the child as he or she grows to adulthood. Sociological studies indicate that those with little or no formal education do not practice preventive health care and there has been a long-time correlation between those with higher education to the amount of preventive health visits. Examples of mindsets are seen in today's dental offices as practitioners hear patients acknowledge that their parents or grandparents had dentures at 30 years of age so they are likely to meet the same fate. Dentists, dental hygienists, and dental assistants are still hearing scare tactics used today by parents. In order to get children to cooperate when visiting the dental office, the parent threatens the child with a "shot" from the dentist if they don't behave. This then results in the adult who avoids the dental office, stating that negative childhood experiences resulted in only seeking dental care in emergency situations.

All of these barriers have created a huge challenge for the health care profession in being able to instill preventive health values and increasing access to all. Although the progression and technology of preventive dental care has increased, the number of consumers retaining their dentition for a lifetime and the challenge to reeducate the patient that has culturally or family-engrained values for little need for oral health care becomes especially difficult. As the factors in barriers to care are numerous and diverse in nature, the solutions for change and elimination are equally challenging and diverse.

Federal and State Programs

Even more costly to society are the expenses associated with oral health problems. The Surgeon General reported that the nation's annual dental bill for the year 2000 was expected to exceed $60 billion. This figure did not include the expenses for medical care related to oral and craniofacial pain (e.g., temporomandibular disorders, trigeminal neuralgia, shingles, or burning mouth syndrome), cleft lips and palates, oral and pharyngeal cancers, the cost of autoimmune diseases, and the cost associated with intentional and unintentional injuries that affect the hands and face. The report also mentioned there would be costs for psychological consequences and costs and other conditions (U.S. Dept. of Health and Human Services, 2000, p. 4).

So where does America stand with facilities providing access to care, funds for consumers needing care, and communities addressing oral health? The American Dental Education Association (ADEA) points out in a 2003 report on improving the oral health status of Americans that the traditional model of oral health delivery, which is the solo practice dentist, is no longer adequate to address the needs of the nation's oral health. Each state also has its own set of laws and regulations, which limit the type of practice settings that can be offered to consumers. They also restrict educated and licensed providers to specific supervision categories, which then limits access to care. Funds allotted to state programs for consumers seeking dental care are also limiting, which means providers like dentists and dental hygienists are not getting reimbursed adequate rates from assistance programs, which limits them from providing dental services. It becomes cost-prohibitive to do business. Oral health has become such an issue that it must be addressed at all levels.

Federal programs have been developed, yet many states and organizations may not be taking advantage of them. The U.S. Department of Health and Human Services has another arm that identifies deficits and develops programs that can be accessed by consumers and providers alike. They are known as the Health Resources and Services Administration (HRSA). Their mission is to improve and expand access to quality health care for all and their goal is to move toward 100 percent access to health care and zero health disparities for all Americans.

Some of the programs that can be found with HSRA are adult and child dental coverage through the Medicaid programs. With the adult program, there may be some dental services that are not provided. It is essential to have preventive care and be able to address existing oral conditions that are in need of treatment. However, because funding must cover millions of adults, these programs must limit the types of services available or that they are willing to pay. Children are also covered under the Medicaid program. For children, Medicaid services are more comprehensive in nature and typically covers a child from birth to 20 years of age. HRSA also addresses providing services in health centers that are federally qualified, which are typically medical facilities. However, HRSA reports that of those qualifying for this program only one in three provide dental services. Medicaid can also reimburse dental services that are provided at a school-based clinic or setting. Many rural areas have schools that include a small health clinic that provides both medical and dental services to children on site. These settings have disappeared over time, yet may be another opportunity for communities to expand access to care.

Another area that HRSA is working on improving is the reimbursement rates for dental services; however, those participating in a Medicaid program must agree to accept the fees established by Medicaid. This is where disparity increases, since the cost of delivering dental care has increased, and Medicaid is not increasing reimbursement rates in correlation. The situation gives rise to decreased provider participation. HRSA is targeting key areas to alleviate the concerns of participating providers, which include streamlining administration, creating a benefit structure, marketing to potential providers, case management to reduce missed appointments, and improved reimbursement rates. Additionally, transportation, parent outreach, and working with Head Start programs and managed care programs are among the issues that require changes if access to care is to improve.

State programs include the State Children's Health Insurance Program (SCHIP). SCHIP is an opportunity for each state to expand access to health and dental services for children. SCHIP was enacted as Title XXI of the Social Security Act in 1997. There are specific criteria set for children to qualify for SCHIP coverage. States can also implement SCHIP as a branch of Medicaid or as a separate program. By having this flexibility it can allow states to bridge a gap and provide more children health and dental coverage. Each state will have a program set up where parents can apply for insurance coverage for their children. For example, some insurance premiums may only cost the family $9.00 per child. This would include dental and medical coverage; although some procedures may not be included in the coverage, families currently without health coverage have the opportunity to be sure their children can get care when needed. As mentioned, each state has designed its own program and it will take some investigation to find more information. However, HRSA has made such programs possible.

It should be mentioned that although many families may meet the criteria to qualify for such programs, many choose not to do so. Reasons are diverse: intimidation, embarrassment, or perhaps unfortunately they are not legally registered in the United States.

Foundation for Patient Education

The material presented in this chapter is done with the intent for each student to begin an understanding of the many facets of dental health education. It is not limited to what is seen in the oral cavity on any given day upon employment in private practice. As a dental hygiene student, it is imperative to fully understand all possible factors that may influence the current oral condition of the patient sitting in the chair. With so many external factors, such as socioeconomic and cultural, that could exceed or equal the internal factors such as systemic disease and oral disease etiology, understanding that there is more to every patient than what is seen clinically will ultimately influence the oral health education provided. As each student learns of the significant facts affecting society as a whole, he or she can assist in the patients' understanding of how to improve their dental health status. The more informed the dental hygienist is about current oral health trends and programs that are available in their state or community, the more they will be able to educate their patients toward improved oral health.

Summary

The oral–systemic link of disease has been growing in acceptance among health care practitioners for nearly 10 years. All health care providers will be responsible for bridging the gap in consumer education if quality of life is to improve for all people. Statistics still indicate that children, older adults, and low-income families are among those most vulnerable to caries and oral diseases. Oral health and general health must parallel each other for an overall improved quality of life. The dental professional must apply the dental hygiene process of care and partner with each patient so that they become responsible for their own health. Risk behaviors play a key role in identifying deficits and excesses in consumers, thus creating an opportunity for the dental professional to change behavior patterns. Medical health care workers can incorporate simple oral health questions to assist in closing the gap between the two fields, and total health is addressed.

Access to care has not improved due to numerous barriers that include socioeconomic status, education, cultural, and financial. Not only is access to care a problem for consumers, it is a problem for health care providers due to low reimbursement rates, funding for facilities, and drawing licensed practitioners to areas in need of health care services.

There are federal and state organizations attempting to alleviate some of the barriers, however, communities will have to play a major role in creating access to care for those residing locally. Programs have been developed to assist major and minor organizations with funding, yet many do not seem to take advantage. Restrictions associated with some of these programs may hinder interest. School-based programs were more prevalent in the past than today and this could be a cost-effective way to increase access.

Critical Thinking

1. What is oral health? Is it the same for everyone?
2. What are the four links of oral disease and systemic disease that are currently most prevalent?
3. How does oral bacteria influence systemic bacteria?
4. How does the dental hygiene process of care play a role in oral health improvement?
5. List some major barriers to dental care.

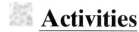 Activities

1. Visit the Health Resources and Services Administration (HRSA) website. Browse the site and see if you can find what programs are available in your state.
2. Identify and discuss specific barriers in your community. (Example: How many public health facilities exist?)
3. Identify and discuss outreach programs for dental care that are ongoing or developing in your community. Who are the key players?
4. Group activity: Develop a program that provides preventive care to children in one elementary school. Will this be a one-day event or will it require more than one day? Include the following:
   - Providers
   - Screening process
   - Oral health education
   - Prophylaxis and sealants
   - Restorative referrals
   - Funding
   - Facilities
   - Public relations

References

American Academy of Periodontology. *Gum Disease increases CRP levels and heart attack risk*, http://www.perio.org, Oral Health Information for the Public, 2003.

Brooke, J. "Periodontal Disease and Pre-term Pregnancy." In *What You Need to Know about Dentistry*. http://dentistry.about.com/library, 2003.

East Sussex, Brighton and Hove Health Authority. http://www.esbhhealth.nhs.uk, 2000.

Henry. Central Statistics Office of Finland 1989. In *Oral Health in the Elderly*. http://www.herkules.oulu.fi, 1995.

Lamster, B., and E. Lalla. "Periodontal Medicine—The Changing Face of Dental Care." *Dimensions of Dental Hygiene* (2004), 10–14.

Offenbacher S., Katz V., Fertik G., et al. "Periodontal infections as possible risk factor for preterm los birth weight. *J. Periodontology*, 1996; 67:1102–1113.

Perry, D. A., P. Beemsterboer, and E. Taggart. *Periodontology for the Dental Hygienist*, 2nd ed. Philadelphia: W. B. Saunders, 2001.

U.S. Census Bureau. *Weinberg, Daniel H. Press Briefing on 2002 Income and Poverty Estimates*. http://www.census.gov/hhes/income02, 2003.

U.S. Department of Health and Human Services. *Oral Health in America: A Report of the Surgeon General Executive Summary*. Rockville, MD: National Institute of Dental and Craniofacial Research, 2000.

World Health Organization. *Oral Health Definition*. http://www.who.int, 1982.

2

Statistics on Oral Health

Objectives

Upon reading the material in this chapter, you will be able to

1. Discuss reasons for the differences in oral health among ethnic populations.
2. Identify trends in disease prevention implemented in private-practice settings.
3. List opportunities for dental education in a community.
4. Discuss national health care concerns as it relates to oral health care.
5. Discuss the cost to implement home oral care recommendations.

Introduction

As mentioned in Chapter 1, the U.S. Surgeon General's Report on Oral Health in America was the first time any official agency addressed the issue so vehemently. The purpose of the report was to point out that not all Americans had the same opportunities to attain optimal oral health and overall well-being. Essentially, Surgeon General Satcher stated that oral diseases were the "silent epidemic" affecting those most vulnerable: poor children, older adults, and members of racial and ethic minority groups. In the fall of 2003, the U.S. Census Bureau reported that nearly 42 million people in the United States were without health insurance and their household income ranged from $25,000 to over $75,000 per year. This not only directly affects those particular individuals; it indirectly affects every consumer in America because the cost of treating oral and health diseases must be assumed somewhere. Having an understanding of how the economy influences health and dental care will assist the student when designing a home care plan that includes proper equipment and oral health aids while keeping within a working budget.

Highlights from the Surgeon General's Report

- Dental caries is the most common chronic childhood disease, 5 times more common than asthma and 7 times more common than hay fever.
- Over 50 percent of 5- to 9-year-old children have at least one cavity or filling, increasing to 78 percent of 17-year-olds.
- Poor children suffer twice as much dental caries as their more affluent peers.
- Uninsured children are 2.5 times less likely than insured children to receive dental care.
- More than 51 million school hours are lost each year to dental-related illness.

Although many communities in the nation advocate water fluoridation, and there have been numerous advances in dental technology, families living in poverty remain unable to seek dental care (Figure 2.1). Race and ethnicity add to the statistics of untreated decay due again to annual income and lack of health benefits (Figure 2.2). From a social standpoint it becomes difficult to understand how a country such as the United States allows such disparities in health, yet young adults are also among those with a high percentage of untreated tooth decay due to low-income levels. Statistics indicate that 46.7 percent non-Hispanic poor adults 18 years and older have a higher percentage of untreated tooth decay than their peers with higher income levels or health insurance, showing a 30.2 percentage of untreated decay. The Mexican American population of poor young adults have 46.9 percent with untreated decay while only 21.9 percent of the same ethnic population with higher income report untreated decay. Thus, untreated decay remains high in those who are unable to pursue appropriate dental care when needed.

Caries is an ongoing disease and the theory of caries transmission is something that must be clearly understood by the health care professional so that it can be articulated to patients throughout one's career. This process is discussed at length in a later chapter.

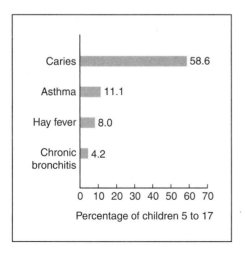

FIGURE 2.1 Dental caries is one of the most common diseases among 5- to 17-year olds. (*Source:* NCHS, 1996, www.hrsa.gov)

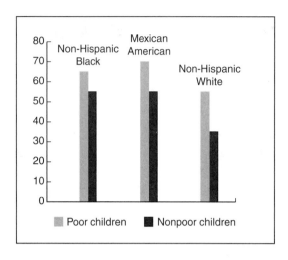

FIGURE 2.2 Poor children aged 2 to 9 in each racial/ethnic group have a higher percentage of untreated decayed primary teeth than nonpoor children. (*Source:* NCHS, 1996, www.hrsa.gov)

Periodontal diseases is the next area reported by Dr. Satcher focusing on the adult population.

- Severe periodontal disease (6 millimeters of attachment loss) affects about 14 percent of adults aged 45 to 54.
- 35 percent of 65- to 74-year-olds have severe periodontal disease, with men affected more than women.
- About 30 percent of adults age 65 or older are edentulous and is higher for those living in poverty.
- Employed adults lose more than 164 million hours of work each year due to dental disease or dental visits.
- For every adult 19 years or older without medical insurance, there are three without dental insurance.

Here again, figures change due to gender and race/ethnicity. Dr. Satcher points out that in every age group a higher proportion of those at the lowest socioeconomic status level have at least one site with attachment loss (6mm or more, Figure 2.3). Gingival diseases are more evident among Mexican Americans (63.6%) than any other ethnic group and early-onset periodontitis is four times more common in males under age 35 than in females.

The data gathered and reported for the U.S. Surgeon General's report indicated that overall, health care in America is severely lacking; the reasons being many, as previously discussed in Chapter 1. Barriers to health care become involved and complicated to address at all levels. However, as a future health care provider, what do these numbers mean?

Statistics are just that, numbers. Yet, they represent the magnitude of oral health problems, whether discussing an individual or a nation. As an oral health care provider it becomes important to understand what these numbers represent. Educating consumers is the most effective avenue for decreasing disease rates and improving oral health status. The dental professional is the first step in accomplishing this overwhelming task.

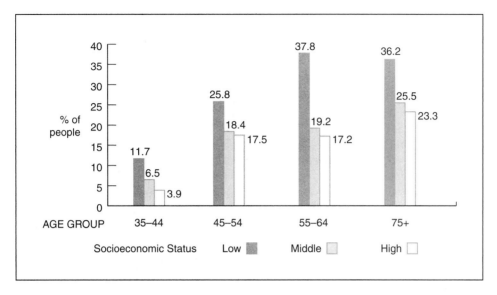

FIGURE 2.3 The percentage of adults with at least one tooth site with 6 mm or more of periodontal attachment loss is greater among persons of low socioeconomic status at all ages. (Adapted from NCHS, 1996, www.hrsa.gov; Burt and Eklund, 1999)

Current Trends in Disease Prevention

Most practitioners and educators would agree that one-on-one education is the best method to get the message to the consumer when it comes to making the difference in oral health, yet it is also a slow and arduous process. Every member in a community will not patronize the same office, and there are a limited number of oral health educators employed in an office that have the opportunity for quality time in order to do so.

During dental hygiene education, students have extended clinic sessions that allow for adequate assessment, treatment planning, education, and debridement. In private practice, the amount of time spent on oral hygiene instructions gets cut to a few minutes. Both situations allow for the clinician to focus on that particular patient's oral condition and need for modification. Making a significant impact in only a few minutes requires background knowledge of oral diseases and high communication skills. Thus, chairside education has a great advantage for the practitioner. There are no interruptions or distractions. The focus remains on one person and what it will take for them to improve their overall oral health. Intraoral cameras have become a great asset, not only from a practice management standpoint, but also from an education standpoint. The original idea behind the development and implementation of the intraoral camera was to be able to have the patient actually see what the dental provider sees during an examination. It was a way for the dentist to validate the need for replacing a restoration or diagnosing the need for a new restoration and a way for the dental hygienist to validate the need for specific hygiene services.

As of recent years, the intraoral camera has become the single best tool for educating the patient on their oral condition and where the focus must be placed in order to improve their condition. The patient is now a partner in his or her own oral health. When the dental hygienist takes an intraoral camera and peruse the oral environment, the patient may find it more difficult to find "reasons" they are not compliant with using a toothbrush and floss. The positive side is that now each time the patient is seen for a regular dental visit, they are able to see the oral health improvement that occurs when compliance is met.

Another positive aspect for using the intraoral camera is for the practitioners themselves. It allows one to actually see areas that may not be seen during a standard intraoral examination. The camera has access to the most distal and lingual aspects of the mouth; areas traditionally accessed only with indirect vision (mirrors) and lighting—not to mention tactile exploring. The dental hygienist can use this visual information to enhance treatment planning and oral health education. The fact that most intraoral cameras can print photos is another tool to show "before and after" conditions of the mouth. Thus, as an education and prevention tool, the intraoral camera can be the dental hygienist's best advocate for getting that all-important message to each patient during their regular dental examinations.

Now take into consideration the magnitude of education required to address oral health to different target populations. For example, how would one undertake oral health education in a school setting? Elementary schools typically have a school nurse assigned to several schools within a particular school district. Oral health education for one individual assigned to several schools is nearly impossible. Thus, many communities will employ the assistance of professionals volunteering their time to educate school children on oral health. Additionally, many dental hygiene programs incorporate community-oriented education during their programs that allow students to become involved at the local level. Here again are two examples of workforces that may be limited to the number of personnel and/or hours to accomplish the task of making a significant impact on oral health among a population of children.

Selecting **target groups,** designing an oral health education program for different age levels, and implementing the education becomes a great task. In a school setting, the environment is not conducive to reevaluating whether your message has been accepted, let alone whether compliance has occurred. The numbers of individuals increases. The oral health educator may be presenting to one classroom of 20 to 30 children, or perhaps an entire grade level, which could increase to 100. Then there could be the school-assembly approach to education, where the entire school is gathered in the auditorium.

For school-based presentations, the simple fact is that repetition aids in ingraining the message. When dental practitioners provide oral health education in a classroom setting, repetition of that message typically does not occur. It's essentially a one-shot chance for making an impact with the children on the importance of oral health, thus the presentation must have aspects that help them retain the message. The age range of the group will depend on how the lesson is designed. Learning levels must be taken into account. For example, if too simple, boredom could occur with older children, yet if the message contains too much technicality by way of verbiage, none of them will know what you are talking about. Therefore, education for larger groups requires more planning and participation to be successful.

Some communities are fortunate to have organizations and funding to employ mobile dental vans. These vans house dental operatories and the equipment to deliver on-site dental treatment. Many of them may be limited to preventive procedures such as screening, prophylaxis, fluoride treatments, and sealants, yet the intention is to access those who may not visit the dental office on a regular basis. This approach to dental care introduces children to dental professionals and, in time, assists in developing a good dental patient.

Another way for approaching oral health education in a community is to participate in health fairs that occur throughout the year. Most cities will hold health fairs that target specific issues, such as breast cancer, or specific populations, such as older adults or children. When local dental professionals, dental schools, and students participate in these activities, it provides the opportunity to disburse oral health information. Many consumers can be approached as to their awareness of oral health and systemic health factors, as well as getting brochures disbursed targeting an aspect of oral health.

Oral health manufacturers oftentimes will assist by donating products that are dispensed during the event. Many of these health fairs offer screenings for cholesterol, blood sugar, and blood pressure, so why not dental screenings? The dental professional certainly can provide a quick visual screening that is noninvasive. Referring the consumer to their dental office helps to improve oral health and systemic health awareness. One area where consumers are lacking in knowledge is systemic health linked to oral health. This topic alone can be presented to consumers as they roam the health fair gathering information.

Here too is another way of educating consumers on oral health. Again, the major disadvantage is that the message is not repeated, and it is not the desired one-on-one education as with a chairside approach. However, oral health education has to occur at all levels. Dental professionals believe that education is key to decreasing oral diseases. Education allows the consumer to change their oral health status. Knowledge on oral diseases allows the consumer to make appropriate decisions regarding their health and how to maintain that health. Thus, it is imperative for the dental professional to understand the magnitude of oral disease and what it will take to make a change. Although many believe changes are made one step at a time, when it comes to dental diseases, one step will not be sufficient. It will take much larger leaps to make a significant impact on the status of oral health.

National Health Care Issues and Oral Health Care

The U.S. Department of Health and Human Services houses the Office of Disease Prevention and Health Promotion. This office is currently working on *Healthy People 2010*, a program designed to promote health objectives for the nation to achieve over the next decade. Scientists created this program as they identified public health priorities. Primary goals for *Healthy People 2010* are first to increase quality and years of health life, and second to eliminate health disparities. *Healthy People 2010* has specific focus areas as well as leading health indicators (Tables 2.1 and 2.2).

With each focus area and each health indicator, those working on *Healthy People 2010* will have to develop strategies to achieve such goals. Goals, of course, are designed to be

TABLE 2.1   Focus Areas for *Health People 2010.*

1. Access to quality health services	15. Injury and violence prevention
2. Arthritis, osteoporosis, and chronic back pain	16. Maternal, infant, and child health
3. Cancer	17. Medical product safety
4. Chronic kidney disease	18. Mental health and mental disorders
5. Diabetes	19. Nutrition and obesity
6. Disability and secondary conditions	20. Occupational safety and health
7. Educational and community-based programs	21. Oral health
8. Environmental health	22. Physical activity and fitness
9. Family planning	23. Public health and infrastructure
10. Food safety	24. Respiratory diseases
11. Health communication	25. Sexually transmitted diseases
12. Heart disease and stroke	26. Substance abuse
13. HIV	27. Tobacco use
14. Immunization and infectious diseases	28. Visions and hearing

Source: U.S. Department of Health and Human Services

broad in scope as true achievement will be difficult, thus the idea of establishing goals. Notice the placement for oral health on the focus list and access to care on the health indicator list. Also notice the types of diseases in the first 10 slots in the focus area list and the health indicators in the first 5 positions. It becomes apparent that one's health habits will influence one's health status, thus the idea behind healthy habits and healthy lifestyles.

The establishment of such a comprehensive disease prevention program can only be done when numerous organizations work together for a commonality.

As presented here, one can see that addressing systemic health and oral health must be done at all levels, nationally to individually. By doing so, tools are provided to all health care organizations to aid in disease prevention and the promotion of health. It falls upon the health professional to take an active role in educating consumers. There is a multitude of ways to accomplish such education, from chairside to whole communities. Improving the oral health status of children and adults will ultimately decrease dental disease. The task remains a large one even with technological advances in dental treatment delivery. It

TABLE 2.2   Leading Health Indicators for *Healthy People 2010.*

1. Physical activity	6. Mental health
2. Overweight and obesity	7. Injury and violence
3. Tobacco use	8. Environmental quality
4. Substance abuse	9. Immunization
5. Responsible sexual behavior	10. Access to health care

Source: U.S. Department of Health and Human Services

will be the grassroots oral health provider such as the dental hygienist that makes an impact on oral health education by getting involved not only with patients that are seen each day in private-practice settings, but participating at a higher level in one's community.

 # Financial Cost Trends of Oral Health and Home Care

For those practitioners who have been working with patients in private-practice settings, the cost of compliance has increased over time, and included many technological changes. The dental professional now has the responsibility to keep up with costs to the consumer and the changes in home care equipment that one may recommend. Let's look at the basics and go from there.

The basic toothbrush used to sell for 50 cents in the 1970s. Now toothbrush manufacturers employ more technology for plaque removal: what works and what works better. Competition among the manufacturers themselves have become a media and clinical trial war. This toothbrush works better than that one because of the bristle design, or because of the way the bristles are constructed and placed on the handle, the number of rows, the direction of the bristles . . . it is endless! What is a professional to do? For that matter what is a consumer to do?

Dental hygienists learn that more than anything; it will be the mechanical removal of bacteria to make the difference in one's oral health. Yet, no matter if you're in a private-practice setting or working in public health, the cost of patient compliance must be taken into consideration. What used to cost 50 cents now costs $5.00! If the patient is of low socioeconomic status, how easily can a $5.00 toothbrush be purchased? But let's go one step further. Currently, most dental professionals will recommend power toothbrushes, not only for design, but also for the mechanics of plaque debridement. Let's face it, power toothbrushes far outweigh manual debridement. They are faster, move at more cycles per minute, and do less damage (abrasion). Therefore, all consumers can benefit from a power brush in some way.

One factor that keeps consumers from purchasing this technology for plaque debridement is the cost. The major manufacturers of toothbrushes produce the rechargeable battery-operated version at a cost of $5–15 to the "high-frequency" version ranging from $40–120. Consider it luck if these devices are found on sale at any time of the year. Those families who are categorized in the low-income bracket will most certainly be unable to spend $120 on a power brush, no matter how much it will improve their oral health and lengthen their lifespan. Spending $5.00 per brush may be enough to strain the budget as it is.

Toothbrushes, of course, are not the only dental items used by consumers. Keep in mind the cost for a tube of toothpaste ($3–6), mouthrinses ($5–9), and dental floss. Summarizing these items for one person can be expensive enough, yet for those on tight budgets and having to supply an entire family it becomes more stressful to comply with oral health recommendations from the dental professional. Table 2.3 lists commonly recommended oral health care items and an approximate purchase price. Thus, it may not be

TABLE 2.3 Samples of Dental Health Care Items and Cost to Consumers.

Dental Care Item	Approximate Cost to Consumer
Manual toothbrush (1)	$ 5.00
Dental floss (1)	1.50
Toothpaste (1-large)	5.00
Mouthrinses w/ fluoride (OTC)	6.00
Power toothbrush (1)	95.00
Water irrigator (1)	55.00
Prescription fluoride (monthly)	25.00
Prescription mouthrinses (16 oz bottle)	20.00

financially feasible for all families or consumers to comply with oral health recommendations at a 100 percent level. Cost factors must be accounted for when designing a home care plan for each patient.

The cost to provide dental care has risen as well and is burdened by the dental professional as well as the consumer. During the early 1980s the cost of a full-coverage porcelain crown was approximately $290. In today's market the cost range is $700 to over $1,000 per crown. Geographic location of dental practices accounts for a lot of the variance in fees charged to consumers. For basic dental hygiene procedures such as scaling, radiographs, and an examination, the costs run anywhere from $95 to $150 per visit. With these fees comes additional cost for restorations, partial dentures, root canals, and more. One never knows what it will take to maintain their dentition. Not to mention the costs of esthetics such as tooth whitening, anterior veneers, and dental implants, which are becoming more popular with time. With nearly 43 million Americans uninsured as of 2003, not many will have the disposable income to cover these costs with regularity. Here again it must be stated that those most vulnerable to decreased oral care will be children. So how can the average consumer and the average family afford appropriate dental health care with rising costs of delivering quality oral health care?

As mentioned in Chapter 1, the number of U.S. families living in poverty has risen to an all-time high as of 2003. Additionally, the number of Americans no longer with health insurance has risen. For example, the cost to provide health care becomes prohibitive to the small business employer (Table 2.4).

The cost for providing health care coverage to employees by employers listed in Table 2-4 are numbers from over a decade ago. It is safe to say that in today's market the cost has risen dramatically, thus employers have not been able to carry health insurance. Also, keep in mind that only three types of trades are presented from the CDC's survey list. Most employers purchase health plans that require the employee to pay an equal amount on an annual basis, termed *matched contributions*. This aspect in itself has financial impacts on those who are categorized in the low-income bracket because it means the net salary decreases. The need to address employer costs as well as consumer costs for health care is something that is not an easy "fix." It is likely to take decades and government leaders to truly determine the best way to provide health care to all.

TABLE 2.4 A Sample of Health Care Premium Costs to Employers.

Type of Establishment	Firm Size (# of employees)	Cost to Employer for Family Health Coverage ($)
Construction	Under 10	850
	100–499	1,148
Retail trade	Under 10	1,065
	100–499	2,143
Services	Under 10	946
	100–499	1,647

Source: U.S. Department of Health and Human Services, 1993 Centers for Disease Control and Prevention

Paying for Dental Care

As private-sector employers decrease health benefits to their employees, the burden becomes the government's. Not only from a national level but also from the state level. Each state, as mentioned, will provide some kind of assistance to those at a certain annual income level. Even so, children may be the only family members to qualify for state assistance, whereas the parents will not; another health care disparity for low-income families. However, keep in mind, as discussed in Chapter 1, a barrier for accessing dental care will be the number of dental practices willing to accept patients covered by state assistance. As new licentiates enter the working environment, they need to be aware that the most common reason dental offices do not participate in state assistance programs is because the

TABLE 2.5 Samples of Reimbursement Rates to Dental Offices for Consumers Covered by a State Assistance Program.

Dental Procedure	Approximate Private-Practice Fee	State Assistance Reimbursement
Periodic examination	$45	$15
Pit and fissure sealants	$25–40	$18–22
Child prophylaxis w/ fluoride	$45–60	$30–40
Adult prophylaxis	$70–95	$30–40
Bitewing x-rays (2 films)	$30–40	$10–15
Full-set x-rays (18 films)	$95–120	$30–45
Root planing 1 quadrant	$120–240	$40–50

Source: Various State Assistance Schedules of Allowances

(*Disclaimer:* The costs featured in this text are only designed to allow the future dental professional to better understand why the number of care providers are scarce in all states, and are not meant to imply an actual reimbursement rate for any single state.)

reimbursement rates for all services are far below the cost to purchase the materials for restorative procedures. It simply does not benefit the provider. Table 2.5 lists some of the reimbursement rates that may take place across many states in the nation.

As depicted, these are but a few procedures that will impact the dental hygienist and the treatment performed. Yet, as mentioned, most private practices cannot afford to participate in these programs because of the cost to deliver oral health care. Additionally, there will be very few communities that will have public health facilities including dental services open for everyone. The cost to a community clinic is not much different than that of a dental practice. There are supplies, overhead costs, employees, billing services, equipment, and a building lease.

Summary

The U.S. Surgeon General's Report in the year 2000 was the first time anyone truly looked at the amount of oral disease in American families. The amount of untreated decay in children is astronomical and something that this country should not be facing, given the amount of technology on dental care delivery and the number of economical ways decay can be prevented. Yet, the fact remains that barriers exist for families when seeking dental care. Socioeconomic status ranks as a high barrier and the number of those living at or below the poverty level has increased dramatically to an all-time high in 2003. Additionally, trends for lack of dental care are still seen in ethnic populations such as Hispanics and African Americans.

A number of goals have been established by national agencies to address dental disease that include cost benefit programs such as community water fluoridation. Creating partnerships allows both national and state agencies to increase the workforce and funds to develop prevention programs that can be easily implemented at a local level in any community.

Oral health education provided chairside in any dental practice must expand into larger programs so that entire communities can become more knowledgeable on how to decrease dental disease and improve oral health. The dental hygienist is a key player in the development of, and leading, oral health education programs. Nationally, the *Healthy People 2010* report identifies focus areas and leading health indicators that plague Americans and develop strategies to decrease all health disparities. This report can be applied to health issues and programs at all levels: from chairside to entire states.

One of the largest barriers for improving oral health is the financial cost of the delivery and payment of dental care. The burden not only lies with employers and the cost for health care coverage but for the dental care provider and the reimbursement rates for those enrolled in a state assistance program. It is not feasible for those in the private sector to accept state assistance reimbursement due to the fact that it will not cover the costs of dental supplies and a workforce to provide such care. This disparity will be a difficult one to improve yet must be addressed by both government and private-sector entities if oral health is to improve in all Americans. Along with dental care delivery costs are those costs to consumers for compliance with oral health home care recommendations. The cost for toothbrushes, mouthrinses, and other oral health aids continues to increase. It becomes more difficult to purchase items that may be more beneficial to one's oral condition. Manufacturers may have to reconsider the cost of these necessary tools for the average consumer.

The issue for optimal oral health is complex to say the least. It will require the work of many over a long period of time to ensure the quality of oral health care delivery and education. Educators will be in short supply as time continues, thus the need for practitioners to seek participation in research, administration, and public health organizations. Expertise in oral health is invaluable to all private and government agencies.

The dental hygiene graduate has numerous opportunities to provide oral health education whether in a private-practice setting, a community group, and a seminar for medical professionals, or designing a program for a community organization. Understanding the importance of health issues affecting consumers from a national perspective can give the dental hygienist broader knowledge for effective dental health education in any environment.

 ## Critical Thinking

1. List some of the key statistics for oral health disparities as highlighted in the Surgeon General's report.
2. Explain how statistics can impact the significance of dental disease.
3. Identify some of the leading health indicators as they relate to the focus areas listed from the *Healthy People 2010* report.
4. List some of the major financial issues to delivering dental care.
5. List some of the financial barriers to patient compliance for home care.

 ## Activities

1. Contact the local health department regarding oral health programs in your area and present these programs for discussion in class.
2. Locate a local dental office that accepts patients covered by state assistance and inquire as to the issues for the dentist participating in the program.
3. Visit the local grocery or drug store and list some of the purchase prices for dental health products. Compare name brands to generic brands.
4. Visit a local public health or dental clinic to observe the health care delivery methods.
5. Group activity: Contact a local health organization such as a hospital or the state or county health department for information on health fairs that may be in the planning stages for your community. Inquire as to being a participant for oral health care by disbursing information and providing oral health education.

References

U.S. Department of Health and Human Services, Centers for Disease Control. *National Center for Health Statistics: National Employer Health Insurance Survey.* http://www.cdc.gov/nchs, 1993.

U.S. Department of Health and Human Services, Office of Disease Prevention and Health Promotion. *Healty People 2010.* Washington, DC, 2000.

3

Nutrition, Lifestyle Trends, Oral and Systemic Health

Objectives

Upon completion of this chapter, you will be able to

1. Develop nutritional recommendations for the pregnant patient.
2. Provide parents of young children with suggestions for dentally healthy meals and snacks.
3. Identify influences and "hot buttons" for food choices for adolescents.
4. Describe the oral effects of obesity.
5. Provide practical meal recommendations for older patients.

Introduction—Nutrition through the Lifespan

In the process of providing dental hygiene care, the dental hygienist has the opportunity and responsibility to identify oral and systemic excesses and deficiencies in nutrition. After identification, the dental hygienist is obligated to make the necessary recommendations and/or referrals to help direct the patient toward total health.

Prenatal Nutrition Education

Nutritional recommendations should begin before the birth of a child. Dental health care professionals may actually be involved in helping to care for the baby's teeth long before the child is seen as a patient. When a pregnant patient is in the dental office, the oral care staff has the opportunity and indeed responsibility to provide information and encouragement on the importance of an adequate diet during pregnancy. While there is an

27

expectation that patients who seek dental hygiene care are also receiving prenatal obstetric care, this may not be the case. The dental hygienist may be the first health care provider to recognize and address prenatal nutritional issues with a pregnant woman.

The initial assessment of the patient will give the first clue regarding her diet. Does she look thin? Does she appear to be overweight? Many women are understandably concerned with the weight gain that accompanies a normal pregnancy. But we need to encourage the patient to not shortchange the unborn child's nutritional needs while watching her weight.

Effects of "Cravings" and Nausea

A pregnant woman's caloric requirements during pregnancy and lactation increase to a greater degree than any other time in her life. The increased caloric needs may trigger cravings and impulsive eating. Some cravings are based on actual need, but if she is craving a chocolate cream pie, it's doubtful that there is a nutrition-based reason. The irregular eating patterns may contribute to increasing the patient's risk of caries and/or periodontal disease. Many expectant women experience bouts of nausea and vomiting. The "queasy" feeling may be relieved by consuming frequent snacks or small meals. Vomiting places potent stomach acids on the dental surfaces. The enamel is at risk of erosion, demineralization, and caries if this is a frequent occurrence. Frequent snacking or eating is another opportunity for an increase in oral acid levels. If the snack is high in **fermentable carbohydrates,** such as the soda crackers that are often recommended, the salivary pH will drop as the bacteria in the woman's mouth begin to utilize this nutrient, contributing to demineralization of the enamel. This process will also increase the plaque accumulation that contributes to gingival and periodontal diseases.

The dental hygienist is responsible for making a determination of the dental effects of frequent vomiting and/or snacking during the intraoral examination and interview of the patient. Observation of enamel erosion, particularly on the incisal or palatal surfaces, should be a clue for the clinician. If the nausea is severe, the woman and her baby may be at risk due to dehydration and nutritional inadequacies, as well as destructive dental effects.

Pregnancy Gingivitis

Pregnant women may also experience an increased risk for gingivitis due to hormonal influences. The hormones don't cause the pregnancy gingivitis, but they contribute to an exaggerated tissue response to plaque (Wilkins, 1999). During the intraoral examination, the clinician must carefully look for hallmark signs of this inflammation, which presents as gingival redness, enlargement, shiny surface appearance, and bleeding with little provocation. Gingival infections may be precursors to periodontal infections. There is a clearly established connection between periodontal infection in the pregnant woman and preterm, low birth weight infants (Darby & Walsh, 2003).

Nutritional Requirements during Pregnancy

Several nutritional components are critical during prenatal development. Protein is especially important for the developing fetus's tissues. Protein is readily available in meats, eggs, and legumes. Minerals, particularly calcium and phosphorous, are required for developing teeth and bones. When the mother's diet is inadequate in these minerals, the reserves in her bones will be tapped. Good sources of calcium include cheese, yogurt, and dark green, leafy vegetables. Phosphorus is obtained from dairy products, meats, and baked goods.

Vitamins A, D, C, and K are also required for the mineralized tissues. Sweet potatoes and carrots are good sources of Vitamin A. Vitamin D can be found in salmon and fortified milk, and is also manufactured by the skin cells when exposed to sunshine. Hot chili peppers, guava, and kiwi are great sources of Vitamin C and may add a little variety to the pregnant woman's diet. Vitamin K is derived from microflora in the gut and from foods such as dark green, leafy vegetables.

Iron is needed for blood cell development and folate for **neural tube development,** and is easily obtained from meat. The pregnant vegetarian can also find available iron in spinach, legumes, and dried apricots. Vegetarians and nonvegetarians are both usually encouraged to take iron supplements during pregnancy in order to ensure adequate amounts for the unborn baby. Comprehensive formulations of prenatal supplements are generally recommended, as levels of some nutrients such as folic acid may be difficult to obtain, even in a good diet.

Chairside Education of the Pregnant Patient

Educating the pregnant patient on the nutritional aspects of her oral health and that of her baby is a vital part of dental hygiene care. When the dental hygienist has identified that the pregnant woman has been experiencing nausea and frequent vomiting, she should be instructed to rinse her mouth with a solution of baking soda and water to neutralize the acid on the teeth. Brushing immediately after vomiting is discouraged, as the enamel is slightly etched and may be damaged by the mechanical action of the bristles. Frequent snacks of noncariogenic foods may ease the nausea and prevent vomiting. The patient may be encouraged to know that most pregnancy nausea subsides after the first trimester. If the patient seems underweight or shows signs of dehydration due to frequent vomiting, her physician should be consulted.

An interview of the pregnant patient will help to evaluate the adequate or inadequate nature of her diet. A **24-hour recall** may be a useful tool to help make this determination. Beginning with the most recent meal or snack, have the patient recall her food intake for the past 24 hours. This is the opportunity for the clinician to educate and motivate the patient on the critical aspects of her nutrition on her baby's health. This is the time to identify the importance of adequate protein, vitamins, and minerals. The patient needs to understand that the myth of "losing a tooth with every pregnancy" is just that—a myth. Some persons still believe that if the mother is not consuming enough calcium the baby will take calcium from the teeth. Dental hygienists know that once the tooth is formed it is not capable of internal calcium withdrawal. If the intake is insufficient, the unborn baby will draw the necessary minerals—calcium and phosphorus—from the mother's bones, not her teeth. The origin of the myth may be the bone loss that will exacerbate a periodontal condition. The patient's socioeconomic situation should be considered when making nutritional suggestions. Lower-cost products such as legumes and **complimentary proteins** such as corn and rice or potatoes and milk will fill the need for protein as completely as expensive meat products will. The dental hygienist should also encourage her patient to take prenatal supplements as recommended by her obstetric care provider.

 ## Infant Nutrition Education

Mothers of breast-fed infants can be encouraged to continue with nutritional intakes similar to those during pregnancy. The caloric and fluid intake should be increased to keep up with the increasing demands of the infant. Prenatal supplements should be continued during breastfeeding as well. Fluoride supplementation for the infant should also be considered and implemented in the early months.

Formula-fed infants will benefit from fluoride as well. The water that is used to mix the formula should be evaluated for fluoride content before the supplemental dosage is determined.

Breast milk and formula contain adequate amounts of calories and nutrients necessary for the infant's growth and development. It is important that the breast-fed infant be allowed to nurse on his or her own schedule in order to regulate the mother's milk production based on the infant's needs. Feeding supplemental bottles of water or diluting formula with more water than required may contribute to nutritional deficits.

Chapter 5 will discuss feeding recommendations that will help in the prevention of early childhood caries (ECC).

 ## Early Childhood Nutrition

Children seem to have a fairly good grasp of what they need to eat and how much. The parent's responsibility is to provide them with healthy food choices and proper amounts. A toddler will choose French fries and deep-fried chicken pieces if given the opportunity. But if the potatoes and chicken are roasted and cut into bite-sized pieces, the child will eat them just as willingly. Parents probably won't even have to dress in a clown suit and makeup to get their little one to eat! Too often, parents are providing food choices to their children that are high in fat, salt, calories, and cariogenic potential. A 2-year-old will surely drink an 8-ounce cola if given the opportunity, but he or she will just as willingly eat lunch with 2% milk if that is what is offered.

Children have fairly high nutritional demands because of their periods of rapid growth. They may need to eat more often than the traditional "3 squares" each day. Parents should be encouraged to provide healthy snack foods that are noncariogenic or low in **cariogenicity.** Some ideas for healthy snacks that are appealing to toddlers and young children are carrot sticks, cucumber slices, sliced cheddar or mozzarella cheese, sliced apples, or celery filled with peanut butter.

Oral hygiene techniques for young children are discussed in Chapter 5.

Adolescent Nutrition Education

The teenage years are marked by a variety of freedoms and choices. Children that were raised in a household where healthy food was the norm and oral health was emphasized may still make unhealthy food choices when they are out of the home. Two factors that may primarily guide the adolescent's food selection are a seemingly insatiable appetite and peer acceptance. These young people are frequently hungry due to increased caloric demands during periods of rapid growth. If the teen is active in sports, the nutritional demands are even higher. It is important to have high-quality, nutritious meals and snacks available for adolescents, but they are out of the parental and adult sphere of influence for much of the day. If their friends are buying soft drinks from vending machines or candy bars from the convenience store on the corner near school, even teens that know better will tend to go along and buy the same unhealthy foods and beverages that their friends purchase.

The dental hygienist has several options available to help encourage teen patients to make good food choices. It is important to identify the area of influence that will most affect teenagers. The clinician should make individualized nutritional recommendations based on the patient's "hot buttons" (motivational factors). Is this an athletic teen that is interested in high performance? Is this a social and outgoing teen that is interested in relationships? Has the patient had previous restorative dentistry that included injections that he or she would prefer not to experience again? Adolescents are capable of participating in informed decision making. When the process of bacterial response to exposure to fermentable carbohydrates and the resultant caries activity is explained, the teen will likely select a bottle of water over a can of soda when thirsty, if preventing cavities is important to him or her. When a competitive swimmer understands that filling his or her stomach with the nutritionally deficient calories found in a candy bar, for example, may result in a loss of energy during a race, the athlete may choose to take an orange to the swim meet to provide a more lasting energy source.

There is an area of adolescent nutrition that should be addressed here. Eating disorders are more common during this stage of life than any other (Darby & Walsh, 2003). **Anorexia nervosa** is the least common among eating disorders, but probably the most well known. The word anorexia means "without appetite," but actually the appetite is suppressed and denied. The classic profile of the patient with anorexia is a white female between 11 and 14 years old, body weight less than 85% of normal, intense fear of gaining weight, distorted body image, obsessive control of weight through diet and exercise, and if menstruation has begun, misses three consecutive menstrual cycles. Purging (deliberate vomiting) may accompany anorexia, but is not a hallmark feature. Anorexia nervosa is a life-threatening condition. The patient may experience diminished resistance to infection, including oral diseases (Palmer, 2003).

Bulimia nervosa may begin in early adolescence, but is more common in college-aged women (Darby & Walsh, 2003). The vast majority of these patients are female. Episodic binge eating and purging are classic aspects of this disorder. Bulimia literally means "ox hunger," which describes the out-of-control appetite these patients experience. They are not typically underweight. Unlike the individual with anorexia nervosa, these patients feel out of control in most areas of their lives. Oral signs of bulimia nervosa include enamel erosion, parotid enlargement, xerostomia, and trauma to the soft palate from inducing vomiting (Palmer, 2003).

The dental hygienist may discover the indications that would lead to the suspicion of these eating disorders, but the actual diagnosis is outside of the realm of practice for the dental office. After communicating observations and concerns to the dentist, recommendations may be made for a referral. This is a delicate situation. The dental team may run the risk of offending the patient with the suggestion of these disorders, but ethically, it would be wrong not to pursue suspicions.

Adult Nutrition Education

An adult's nutritional needs are more static than those of a growing child. Most adults in this country have a tendency to consume more calories than they need. Even a small number of calories, say 100, beyond the individual's daily need, will add up and result in a gradual weight gain. The number of Americans overweight or obese has increased in dramatic proportions over the last 20 years (CDC, 2004). Obese people in the United States (those with a **body mass index** at or above 30), are numbered at around 44 million, with an additional 6 million people over their desirable weight by 100 pounds or more (see Figure 3.1). Obesity contributes to many systemic conditions, several of which have oral health consequences.

Diabetes is steadily increasing along with weight gain in the American public (see Figure 3.2). Diabetics are at increased risk of periodontal disease and other oral infections. Heart disease, high blood pressure, and cancer are also linked to obesity (CDC, 2002).

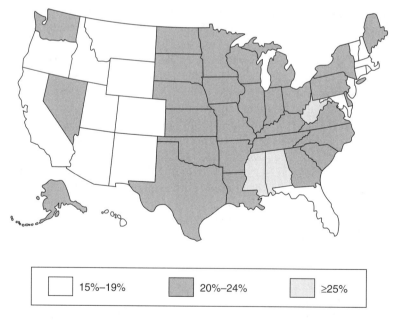

15%–19%   20%–24%   ≥25%

FIGURE 3.1   Distribution of obesity in the United States. (*Source:* CDC National Center for Chronic Disease Prevention and Health Promotion, 2002)

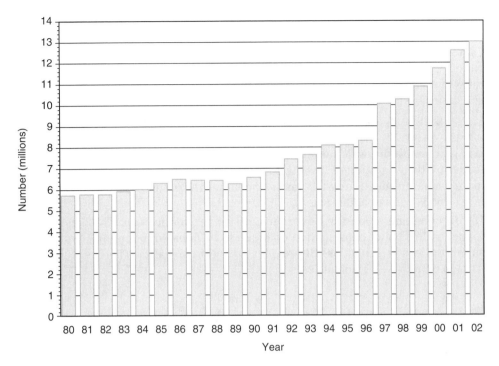

FIGURE 3.2 Number of persons with diagnosed diabetes in the United States, 1980–2002. (*Source:* CDC National Center for Chronic Disease Prevention and Health Promotion, 2004)

The dental hygienist must be able to recognize nutritional excesses that are contributing to the patient's weight gain. The 24-hour nutrition recall is a tool for chairside assessment and evaluation of the patient's eating habits. It is not an accurate representation of the individual's true nutrition patterns (Palmer, 2003). A 4- to 5-day journal or food diary that includes one weekend day is more accurate. The clinician should then be capable of recognizing patterns and providing the patient with recommendations that will assist the patient in establishing more healthy eating habits. When the dental hygienist recognizes nutritional excesses and patterns that are particularly destructive, or when a patient is not responsive to suggestions, a referral to a nutrition professional should be considered.

Adults, like patients of all ages, should be encouraged to eat a well-balanced diet that includes all of the necessary nutrients. Even though many adults overconsume calories, they may be lacking in key nutrients as well as antioxidants and fiber. Following the USDA/Health and Human Services dietary guidelines is a good way to ensure a healthy diet:

Eat a variety of foods. This helps to minimize the risk of inadequate vitamin and mineral sources.

Maintain a healthy weight. If you are underweight, you should consume more high-quality calories; if overweight, consume fewer calories.

Choose a diet low in fat, saturated fat, and cholesterol. This helps to lower calories and also helps the patient become more aware of the types of fat they are selecting.

Choose a diet with plenty of vegetables, fruits, and grain products. This is for a variety of benefits, including the interest provided by their colors, flavors, and textures, but fiber may be one of the most important assets provided by vegetables, fruits, and grains.

Use sugars in moderation. Sugars quickly increase the caloric intake. The frequency of sugar exposure adds to the patient's oral disease risk as well.

Use salt and sodium in moderation. Persons at risk for hypertension are directly affected by their salt intake. Salting food also seems to become a habit that requires more and more added to satisfy taste. Encourage the patient to try to enjoy the flavors of the foods without added salt.

If you consume alcoholic beverages, do so in moderation. The benefits of light-to-moderate alcohol consumption continue to be debated, but no one would argue in support of heavy alcohol use. It provides non-nutritive calories and may block the utilization of other valuable nutrients.

Nutrition Education for the Older Patient

Overall caloric needs are lessened in older adults, but some key nutrient requirements are increased. It is not uncommon to discover nutrient deficiencies in older people. Some of the oral manifestations of deficiencies in the B-complex vitamins, for example, include atrophic glossitis, angular chelitis, and complaints of a burning sensation of the tongue (Palmer, 2003).

There are several reasons for nutritional deficits in older patients. Many adults believe that a balanced diet is something required only by growing children and pregnant women, and therefore may not seriously consider basic food guidelines. Older adults may have a lessened appetite that is related to their diminished senses of taste and smell. The appetite may also be reduced due to pathology. A limited income may cause patients to feel like they can't afford to prepare complete meals. There may be issues such as loneliness and a lack of interest in preparing foods and eating alone. Alcoholism may also be a factor to consider. The older patient may be practicing outdated methods of food preparation that don't preserve the nutrients as well as more modern methods. They may have dental problems including missing teeth or ill-fitting dentures, contributing to the selection of easy to chew foods that may be nutritionally lacking. Another common oral problem for older patients is **xerostomia.** A dry mouth can make chewing and swallowing difficult. Finally, intestinal and digestive disorders may prevent the absorption of nutrients.

The dental hygienist can identify possible causes of the older patient's nutritional deficiencies, and may be able to provide practical suggestions. The individual should understand that a balanced diet is necessary for all ages (refer to the USDA/HHS guidelines). The dilemma of diminished appetite due to diminished taste and smell senses may be addressed by encouraging the patient to purchase prepared frozen meals. It is often difficult to plan and prepare a meal without an appetite that stimulates interest, so a prepackaged meal may be a practical solution. If the appetite is diminished due to a condition or pathology, a consultation with the patient's physician may be in order.

Many older patients live alone and may find preparing and eating meals alone to be an unpleasant experience. The dental hygienist will want to be aware of senior nutrition programs in the area. Some programs deliver meals to seniors while others provide daily meal service in a community facility. This solution may also apply to the elderly patient that is on a limited income or prepares food using styles of preparation that contribute to a loss of nutrients (such as boiling vegetables or deep-frying foods). These programs are usually government-funded and are mandated to uphold high nutritional standards, so the dental hygienist can be confident that the patient is benefiting from well-balanced meals.

The older patient needs to understand that a balanced diet doesn't need to be expensive. Some practical ideas can be communicated that will enhance the diet. Purchasing seasonal fruits and vegetables is always more cost effective than purchasing the produce that is out of season, for example. Fresh carrots, onions, celery, and lean beef will make a beef stew for several meals that will usually cost less than the canned alternative and may be more appetizing as well.

The older alcoholic patient may be consuming an abundance of calories in the beverage, but probably won't be eating a balanced diet. Two ounces of 86 proof liquor contains about 137 calories. In addition to inadequate intake, alcohol may prevent the metabolism of necessary nutrients (Palmer, 2003). Simple meal ideas may be suggested, as well as nutritional supplements such as Ensure. Supplements and liquid meal replacements may also be beneficial to the patient with dental problems that are impairing adequate mastication. This can be a temporary solution, however, the individual will want to have the necessary dental treatment completed in order to remedy the problem.

The patient with a digestive disorder would benefit from a consultation between the dental hygienist and the physician. The physician may be aware of the problem and the nutrients affected.

Xerostomia is common in older patients. It has many causes, including radiation therapy in the head and neck region, Sjögren's syndrome, and as a side effect in over 500 medications (Darby & Walsh, 2003). The individual with xerostomia may have difficulty chewing and swallowing because of insufficient saliva. This may cause the patient to choose moist, soft foods, which may be high in calories and cariogenic effects. The dental hygienist can suggest soft, moist, **nutrient-dense foods** such as cottage cheese, scrambled eggs, soups, and yogurt. Frequent sips of water with meals will aid difficulty in swallowing. It should be emphasized that sipping water is preferred over larger drinks of water to avoid causing the patient's stomach to become full of water, possibly inhibiting adequate food consumption.

The Fast Food Influence

"Fast foods" have had a profound effect on the diet and nutrition of American consumers, one that cannot be overlooked by the dental health care professional. The concept of being able to purchase food that has been prepared by someone else without even having to leave our cars fits into the busy lifestyles of many Americans. In his book *Fast Food Nation*, Eric Schlosser reveals that Americans spend more money on fast food than on higher education. Fast food spending exceeded $110 billion in 2001. Americans aren't selecting these foods based on their nutrient levels, they are selecting them because they are convenient, inexpensive, and they taste good. (Or they value the toy that comes with the "fun meal.")

Of course, the problem is that with all of these billions that are being spent on fast food come billions of excess calories. The hamburger restaurant companies utilize sauces heavily laden with fats, foods cooked in fat, and sweet beverages that are irresistible to many people. Add a multibillion dollar marketing plan, some movie endorsements, and the value of "super-sizing" and the result is inevitable; there are more obese Americans now than any other time in history.

An observable outcome of this trend is that children in this country are getting more obese and less fit every year. Dangerous blood pressure and cholesterol levels are being observed in younger children, while the incidence of **Type II diabetes** continues to climb. Obese children are predisposed to obesity as adults, and will experience an increased risk of not only diabetes, but also colon cancer, stomach cancer, breast cancer, arthritis, heart disease, high blood pressure, strokes, and infertility (CDC, 2002).

The trend in America's "fast food addiction" seems to be ongoing, so the dental hygienists has the opportunity to provide patients with guidelines to help them make healthier fast food choices, some of which include:

1. Restaurants provide nutritional information upon request. Encourage patients to compare their favorite franchise restaurant foods. Consumers may be surprised to discover that chicken nuggets are higher in fat than hamburgers.

2. Encourage individuals to order small- or regular-sized sodas. Super-sizing adds hundreds of extra calories (310 in a 32-ounce soft drink) that readily convert to stored fat. Some restaurants provide water at little or no cost. Reduced-fat milk is another option.

3. No matter how great the "bargain," encourage the patient to not super-size the french fries. They are a treat that can enhance the burger meal, but not too many people really *need* that many fries. The super-size fries at McDonald's is a serving that is three times larger than the serving size offered in 1972.

4. Encourage patients to order their burgers without mayonnaise or other oil-based sauces. These do add moisture and a pleasant oral sensation, which may be missed if eliminated. Suggest requesting mustard, ketchup, extra pickles, lettuce, and/or tomatoes to add moisture.

5. Grilled chicken breasts are an option in many franchise restaurants. They are a lower-fat alternative to hamburgers.

6. Consider a side salad instead of fries to accompany a burger. Suggest that the patient try seasoning the salad with a squeeze of lemon juice, a dash of vinegar, a sprinkling of pepper, or a small amount of dressing.

7. Patients that consume foods from fast food restaurants frequently should be encouraged to seek alternatives for convenient meals. Preplanning will save time, money, and unnecessary calorie excesses. A peanut butter sandwich on whole wheat bread and an

apple will travel well, won't need to be refrigerated for a long period of time, and will provide a nutritious, satisfying lunch for the busy patient.

Patients will benefit from the awareness and attentiveness of the dental hygienist to their nutritional needs. The dental hygienist may be the health care professional that has "just the right thing" to suggest that may provide positive changes in their nutritional behaviors and overall health.

 # Summary

In the process of providing dental hygiene care, the dental hygienist must recognize the oral and physical signs and symptoms of nutritional excesses and deficiencies. Nutritional needs vary through the lifespan. Food choices are made out of habit, convenience, or preference. Some of these choices may have detrimental effects on the patient's oral and total health.

The pregnant patient is responsible for the nutritional needs of two people. Pregnancy issues such as morning sickness and cravings may contribute to the patient making food choices that aren't the best for her or her baby. The dental hygienist needs to be able to recognize the signs of damage to the teeth from vomiting or from frequent snacking, and make the appropriate recommendations.

There are key nutrients that are required during pregnancy. The dental hygienist has the opportunity to serve as another health care provider that has concern and knowledge that will benefit both the pregnant patient and the baby. Utilize the dental hygiene visit as a chance to teach or remind the patient about what those key nutritional needs are and some of the sources of them.

Breast milk and formula are both adequate sources of most nutrients for meeting the requirements of infants. The dental hygienist must know the amounts of fluoride contained in the area's water in order to recommend the correct fluoride supplement levels, if the area water contains insufficient amounts of this necessary mineral.

The parents of toddlers will appreciate suggestions for healthy snacking. The dental hygienist can also encourage the parent to provide quality foods, being wary of the over-consumption of soft drinks, salt-laden foods, and fried foods. The adolescent patient has high nutritional demands as well as peer influences to consider. The dental hygienist can discover the teen's areas of interest in order to help motivate the individual to make wise food choices for oral and total health. The fast food influence is a particular concern for all patients. Dental hygienists should have practical alternative ideas for individuals that frequently consume fast food products.

Adhering to the guidelines for a healthy diet that are provided by the USDA/Health and Human Services will make it easier for patients to consume adequate nutrients and avoid harmful excesses. These guidelines should be understood by the dental hygienist and utilized in his or her nutrition recommendations. Serious excesses or deficiencies require the services of licensed nutrition experts.

Critical Thinking

1. Identify the key nutrients required by a woman during pregnancy. Name at least two sources of each nutrient for vegetarian and nonvegetarian patients.
2. Identify the medical conditions that are associated with obesity. Which one has a direct oral link?
3. List the guidelines for a healthy diet that were developed by the USDA/Health and Human Services.

Activities

1. Interview a pregnant woman to discover her eating habits. Begin with a 24-hour recall of her diet, and then ask her to keep a 4- to 5-day journal, tracking *everything* that she eats or drinks. Identify excesses or deficiencies in her diet, and then develop a plan to help her modify it if necessary.
2. Interview an older patient to discover his or her eating habits. Begin with a 24-hour diet recall, and then a 4- to 5-day journal that includes meal times and situations. Identify excesses, deficiencies, or patterns that may be harmful. Provide suggestions as needed.
3. Visit a fast food restaurant. Ask to see the nutrition information provided for the food products that are sold in that restaurant. Develop menus for three meals, each providing the consumer with a balance of nutrients and is below 700 calories.

References

Centers for Disease Control, National Center for Chronic Disease Prevention and Health Promotion. *Data and Trends, Diabetes Surveillance System, Prevalence of Diabetes.* http://www.cdc.gov/diabetes, 2004a.

Centers for Disease Control, National Center for Chronic Disease Prevention and Health Promotion. *Overweight and Obesity Health Consequences.* http://www.cdc.gov/nccdphp/dnpa, 2002.

Centers for Disease Control, National Center for Chronic Disease Prevention and Health Promotion. *Overweight and Obesity, Obesity Trends.* http://www.cdc.gov/nccdphp/dnpa, 2004b.

Darby, M. L., and M. M. Walsh. *Dental Hygiene Theory and Practice*, 2nd ed. Philadelphia: W.B. Saunders, 2003.

Palmer, C. A. *Diet and Nutrition in Oral Health.* Upper Saddle River, NJ: Prentice Hall, 2003.

Schlosser, E. *Fast Food Nation/The Dark Side of the American Meal*, Boston, MA: Houghton Mifflin, 2001.

Wilkins, E. M. *Clinical Practice of the Dental Hygienist*, 8th ed. Philadelphia: Lippincott, Williams & Wilkins, 1999.

4

Communication Styles

Objectives

Upon reading the material in this chapter, you will be able to

1. Define active listening.
2. Identify one's own communication style.
3. Discuss methods for building communication skills.
4. Design effective handouts and visual aids.
5. Identify effective learning environments.

Introduction

Communication is learned very early in life. Toddlers learn to communicate by pointing to something they want, making noises, and eventually sounding out words heard from parents. Once their vocabulary increases, children put sentences together with a higher degree of complexity, and eventually through education, sentences become paragraphs, pages, and stories that have significance and structure. Communication is done in various forms: nonverbal or body language, verbal, visual, and written. Effective communication attempts to deliver a specific message concisely. Communication requires that the communicator not only deliver the message, but hear a message.

Listening is another skill often overlooked as an important tool for effective communication. Yes, hearing someone speak on a subject of interest is great; however, really hearing the intended message is something different. How often do you see or are a participant in an argument? Arguments occur between individuals because each person is attempting to make the other understand or accept their viewpoint. Yet, is each one listening to the other? Active listening is designed to make sure one person understands what the other person is actually saying. Understanding how to use active listening will assist in the building of effective communication. When the dental hygienist has a message on the condition of a patient's oral health, it will be important that that message be conveyed in a way that the patient is aware of its significance. Communicating effectively will ensure that the dental hygienist is doing everything he or she can to get their message across and improve their patient's oral health.

Listening

Many do not realize that hearing someone talk and listening to them are two different things. Remember the children's game "Telephone"? The first person whispers a phrase or statement to the second person, and so on down the line. By the time the phrase got to the last person who verbalized what was heard, it was nowhere near how it began. Thus, hearing can be different than listening.

To improve listening skills and become a good listener, it is imperative to know what was stated. How often do you find yourself being interrupted while in a conversation with another, or find yourself interjecting your thoughts and opinions before the other person is finished with their statement? It happens all the time to everyone. Thoughts are developing into statements during a conversation, and we're afraid that if we don't say it now, we'll forget what we wanted to say, so we interrupt with "but . . . but. . . ." Without fully listening to the other person and allowing them to finish their ideas and statements, complete understanding of what is being said does not occur.

What affects a person's capacity for listening? Numerous things will influence how one listens to a speaker, instructor, or their own child. For example, if the subject matter is not interesting to the listener, how much will they really hear? Is it a new subject? Is it something truly of interest that the listener wants to learn about? Is it important? Does the speaker or listener speak a different language? Most often listeners will hear only bits and pieces based on key words that peak their interest. The rest of the topic is placed on a shelf. Another example may be that the speaker is of interest because of their education, experience, or speaking talent. Other things that affect listening may be that the message is buried in so much other material it is hard to extract by the listener or perhaps the room or environment is distracting. Is the speaker or listener trying to multitask during the conversation? If a student, take a look around the classroom. Are there windows? Do other students or people noisily pass the door? Can telephones or conversations be heard? These things must be considered when designing a good listening environment, or better yet a good teaching environment. As a parent or spouse, how often are you involved with household chores while a family member needs your attention as a listener? External factors can most certainly influence the listener and perhaps distort the message. Upon better understanding of what is required as a listener, anyone can improve on eliminating identified external factors.

There are also internal factors that will affect listening, for example, the listeners' perception of the statement, preconceived opinions, emotions, their own experience with the subject matter, their education, or whether or not they even like the person speaking.

When people have a strong conviction or belief on a specific topic, emotions can block what one person is attempting to communicate to the other. Gender differences in communication and listening styles have been an area well studied and written about.

As presented, there are many factors influencing listening, which will then influence communication. For the dental hygienist, it will be beneficial to understand what influences listening so communication can be improved when working with patients, colleagues, coworkers, and employers. Quality communication skills will ensure that the accuracy of the message is received.

Active Listening

What does *active listening* mean? Active listening is intended to focus on whom you are listening to, whether it's an instructor, a patient, an employer, a colleague, or a friend. The listener should be able to repeat what the speaker has stated in his or her own words. It's not how the listener *interprets* what they have heard, only what the speaker has stated. By being able to repeat exactly what was said, the listener is clearer on what was heard. This does not mean the listener has to agree with the statement or interpret its meaning, only that the statement was understood correctly.

The benefits to active listening are (1) the listener is forced to listen attentively, (2) it helps to avoid misunderstandings because the listener must confirm what was stated, and (3) many times people tend to say more. For example, when active listening techniques are used in conflict resolutions, it helps to alleviate each person contradicting or denying the other. Eliminating contradiction and denial during arguments allows the problem to be solved effectively.

Most students and educators would agree that listening is critical to the relationship of the educational process. Educators want and need to be heard if they are to teach effectively, and students need to be able to listen if they are going to learn effectively. In a child's education, they need to know that the teacher cares about them. This provides motivation to learn, as they know the teacher will be happy. In adult education, adults bring life experience into the learning environment. Mutual respect then becomes a motivation to learn the subject well. Active listening skills play a significant role in both of these learning arenas.

As the dental hygiene educator for patients, it will benefit the professional relationship by employing the same active listening skills discussed. Each dental consumer is unique and brings his or her own dental history. During dental hygiene school, students are taught how to teach oral health education to each patient based on their oral condition at that time. Often students will employ the same exact brushing and flossing philosophy to every patient when it might benefit the student to identify current techniques that are already working well for that patient. Did the dental hygiene student *listen* to what the patient had to say about previous dental experiences? Or did they only *hear* certain aspects of the story? There may be some bias in what the dental hygiene student hears from the patient as they already have a planned routine.

Perhaps the following scenario took place during a clinic session:

DH student: How have you been doing with your oral hygiene since the last visit?

Patient: Okay, I can't seem to get the hang of using the floss, though.

DH student: How often are you brushing per day now?

Patient: Two, sometimes three, depending on what I eat that day, or what time I go to bed.

DH student: Are you using the fluoride rinse at night as recommended?

Patient: Sometimes.

DH student: Well, today we are going to go on to the next area and reevaluate the area done last visit.

Some things to consider:

1. Did the student clarify anything said by the patient?
2. Did the student listen to what was stated?
3. Is it apparent the student had a plan and her questions were routine in nature?
4. Was the student interested in the patient's answers?
5. What kind of modification can the student provide, without listening to the patient's answers?

Without attentively listening to what was being stated, how can the dental hygiene student make changes in patient motivation? Patient compliance? The patient won't feel as though anyone cares whether or not flossing or fluoride rinses are used, so why bother. If the clinician does not use active listening skills, the patient perception may be that the dental hygienist is apathetic to their motivation and compliance. The patient is not getting the attention deserved.

As the dental hygiene student or the new graduate becomes more comfortable with a one-on-one relationship with patients, it is likely that *feedback* occurs during conversations of oral health. Feedback will employ questions that the listener will use to clarify the statements being made by the speaker. This approach likely occurs without notice during many conversations under numerous circumstances and environments.

The following may be a typical conversation between the dental hygienist and a patient:

DH: So Mr. H, how have you been doing with your flossing since the last visit?

Mr. H: Well, it's not something I like.

DH: Does this mean you are not flossing?

Mr. H: I really can't find the time to fit it in my schedule.

DH: When are you flossing?

In this example, the dental hygienist is not repeating the statements made by Mr. H, word for word; rather, she is asking a question to clarify the answers made by Mr. H.

How can the dental hygienist employ active listening skills to the daily appointment? Using some of the requirements already discussed, some ideas to begin the improvement process might include:

- Repeating what was said to gain a better understanding.
- Clarifying concerns and questions to improve the patient–clinician relationship.
- Restating the statement so that the patient feels understood and cared about.
- Providing feedback to the statement made in the form of a clarifying question.

So if we use the conversation above and incorporate active listening, it might transpire like the following:

DH: So Mr. H, how have you been doing with your flossing since the last visit?

Mr. H: Well, it's not something I like.

DH: You state that you don't like flossing, correct? Can you explain exactly what you don't like about it?

Mr. H: I really can't find the time to fit it in my schedule.

DH: You say that you can't fit it in your schedule; can you tell me what part of the day gives you more time for yourself?

By incorporating active listening techniques into the dental health education of patients, the dental hygienist will become more effective in communication. Realizing that listening plays a significant role in communication will ensure the accuracy of the message.

The Learning Environment

Oral health education can take place in a variety of settings. Yet, the professional providing the education will want to be sure they know what an environment may present and be ready to work with it or around it. When entering an elementary school classroom, the teacher has taken great care to design the room with educational materials that enhance the classroom, initiate questions from the children, and draw attention and maintain interest using bright colors and shapes. In adult education, the classroom becomes very functional: technology is used by way of computers, Internet sources, and perhaps journals and large reference texts. Additionally, when the dental professional enters a community environment, the surroundings could be that of a hospital conference room or a community center.

When planning a dental health seminar, it is wise to know ahead of time what the environment presents. If the educator needs technology and the assigned room does not provide for computer links, is the educator prepared with another version of his or her material? Is the room too large for a group of 20? Large rooms that may not have carpet or doors will mean echoing and noise coming in from outside. Is the room too small for a group of 50? Small rooms may lend themselves to a feeling of claustrophobia for some, or become too "stuffy" because the air does not circulate well. In many cases, the attendees become tired and drift off to sleep. Are there windows that will allow people to see in as well as out? This can cause a distraction for those attending the seminar. How about lighting that is too bright or too dark? If providing the attendees with a handout and presenting the information on slides, are the lights too dim if someone wants to read or write? All of these factors must be considered when designing an oral health education presentation or seminar, as they will influence the attendee's ability to listen attentively, or hear the speaker.

When a patient sits in the dental operatory and the dental hygienist is providing oral health education, do other staff members enter the room? Do they interrupt and ask questions? Are there children accompanying a parent? Are the noises from the rest of the office so loud that other conversations can be overheard? Is the office music too loud, causing voice volumes to increase during conversation? Education in the dental office is an important factor for improving patient motivation and compliance. When there are too many distractions in the environment, the patient may not process the information being received with a great degree of accuracy.

No matter the environment, the oral health educator will want to consider how to effectively get the message across to the recipient. Be aware of the learning environment and make the necessary changes in the presentation. By doing so, the educator can be assured they are addressing factors that may influence the learning opportunities of those they are educating.

Learning Styles

As previously mentioned, children and adults have different ways of learning. The five senses tend to play key roles with remembering material that is presented in different formats or environments. The same holds true for dental consumers seen each visit whether for a comprehensive examination or their annual dental hygiene appointment. As a health care provider, education is significant for improving oral health. Therefore, the provider will want to use more than one method of teaching to ensure that the patient can learn what is essential to improve or maintain oral health.

Many consumers are ***auditory learners.*** Auditory learners learn best by hearing information. This also means that they are able to remember best by hearing everything explained to them orally. Some of the characteristics of auditory learners identified by Penn State University at the York Campus Learning Center may include:

- The ability to remember accurate details in a lecture or conversation.
- Strong language skills and a well-developed vocabulary.
- Strong communication skills and the ability to articulate clearly.
- The ability to carry on interesting conversations.
- The ability to learn a foreign language easily.
- The ability to hear tones and rhythms and play a musical instrument.
- Articulate exactly what they mean during a conversation.

When preparing an educational topic for auditory learners, the presenter will want to make sure that everything is explained with enough detail. Many educators forget that not everyone understands what is being discussed. This may be due to a lack of detail or examples. Educators in all arenas become very familiar with their subject matter, and can skip important aspects that may assist the auditory learner in learning or remembering the material.

Visual learners make up about 40 percent of all learners. They learn by seeing pictures or print. Visual learners must be able to see the material then write the words. The use of colors may also influence the retention and learning of material. Words heard or read by the visual learner are processed into a mental image and recalled later when needed (Robledo, 2004). Print learners think in words and learn to read quickly. Rita Dunn, director of the Center for the Study of Learning and Teaching Styles at St. John's University in New York, has conducted research indicating that when a child's learning style is accommodated, their academic performance is significantly increased. This finding can be applied for adult visual learners as well.

Some other characteristics of visual learners will include:

- Easy memorization of charts and graphs.
- Easily visualizes what the speaker may be describing.
- Are able to make "videos" of the information they read with detail.
- Have strong spatial skills.
- Play close attention to body language and facial expressions.
- Are aware of aesthetics, visual media, and the beauty in art objects.

Upon developing dental health education material, whether for the patient in the chair, a group of colleagues and community organizations, or the elementary classroom, the dental professional will want to incorporate techniques that address the learning styles previously discussed. When using photos or slides, be aware that the text explains the image. When using text, be aware that descriptive terms or phrases are included to provide a mental image. These tips will assist in effectively communicating the oral health message.

Using Learning Materials

Any educator wants to make sure that the information being presented is remembered and perhaps a future resource for those attending any seminar or class. *Handouts* and *outlines* are a way to disburse the basics of such material. Handouts are a way to ensure that the people attending the presentation will remember what was said as about 90% of what is heard is forgotten within 24 hours (Bull, 2003).

At first glance, any handout looks simple in nature, as if it takes no time at all to put one together. However, a quality handout can take hours for some. There are many things educators will want to consider before creating a handout. Speakers will often give some background information on themselves, and if presenting scientific information there are citations that need to be included or perhaps research methods.

There are visuals and graphics that may be required to substantiate the material being presented, or perhaps visuals that will add humor. Identifying the purpose of the handout

- Color scheme
- Graphics: photos, drawings, charts, tables
- Amount of information: high points, all material
- Text: font style, font size, color, bold or italic
- Page count
- Space for notes
- Resources: cited works, references, Internet sites

FIGURE 4.1 Considerations to include in a quality handout.

will assist in its creation. Essentially, the handout is a synopsis of the entire presentation. Or perhaps it's a synopsis of a research paper or chapter from a text. They are one way to provide additional information or data to what is being verbalized by the educator. Figure 4.1 provides some ideas that can be included in any handout to increase the quality of what is being given to attendees of any class or seminar.

Savvy speakers will use technology in the presentations whenever possible. The handout can reflect such technology as well. Most computer software programs will have a presentation or handout program built in. This makes the creation of handouts and presentations much easier for both the novice and seasoned educator. Many are familiar with Microsoft PowerPoint. This allows any educator to create a slide presentation as well as a handout that will match each slide created. Animation can also be included as it can add interest to the seminar. No matter the type of software on any computer, there are also many websites that assist in the creation of a quality handout that can be a good source of reference (Appendix D). Once the purpose of the handout is identified, its creation will be easier and provide the learner with information that augments the subject of education.

When the dental hygienist educates a patient, one of the most used tools in that education is the use of *visual aids*. Remember that the average dental consumer is unfamiliar with terms used to describe their conditions: gingiva, dentition, alveolar bone, caries, and so on. In order to help the patient understand what is being described, the dental hygienist has the use of flipcharts, brochures, photos, oversized models, or perhaps posters displayed in the operatory. Visual aids such as these provide support for the discussion at hand. Handing a patient a brochure and asking them to read through it without providing a verbal synopsis of the brochure may not ensure that the message is being understood correctly. Between verbalizing the information and providing a visual aid, the dental hygienist is addressing both aspects of auditory and visual learning styles.

Humor is another way to "lighten" the topic of discussion. Humor is often used in public speaking to engage and entertain an audience (Audrieth, 1998). Oftentimes, it helps the audience remember the topic or breaks up monotony. Anyone can use humor when they have to communicate to a group or an individual. It may assist in the motivation of the audience, whether it's one or many. Humor can be used in the form of an anecdote (any interesting event) or as simple as a joke. Some may find incorporating famous quotes or quips help in building rapport, trust, and ease between them and their audience. A fine line may exist between humor and its use in a serious situation, thus the educator will want to take this into consideration.

Most often, the patient is apprehensive about their dental appointment in the first place. Children especially can have a fear of the unknown, and when seated in the dental chair, all the large equipment and aseptic surroundings can be daunting and overwhelming. Humor can be an excellent way to capture attention. The use of funny stories that can be related to the topic of education can assist in the patient remembering what was discussed. Humor is also a way of building good rapport with new patients as well as those who are established in the practice. Creating a "user-friendly" environment assists in making any dental appointment a more pleasant experience.

Teaching/Learning Techniques

Previously mentioned were two ways people learn: auditory and visual. Additionally, was the learning environment or surroundings in the room or venue, or perhaps just the dental operatory. Techniques of teaching are something educators will want to consider in order to be effective in presenting a message. For example, when in the classroom, the teacher often uses *lecturing* as the technique of choice to present information to students. This information may be enhancing a text or research article. Lecturing is defined as an "informative talk." Thus the teacher is presenting a certain volume of information to the audience (students). During lectures, some discussion takes place between the audience and the lecturer, yet it does not allow for a lot of interaction other than that.

Another teaching technique is when the teacher breaks the audience up into *small groups*. Small groups allow the audience to discuss topics as individuals and as a whole class. This format also allows for more interaction between members of the audience, and perhaps more interaction between the audience and the teacher, as the teacher has the opportunity to walk around and visit each group.

Other interactive methods for teaching and learning include the "over-the-shoulder" demonstration. In a dental hygiene program, the instructor often walks around the lab or clinic and observes the students progress, then can assist their technique by demonstration. When providing dental health education, the dental professional may be in an elementary school classroom and walk around assisting the children in the task requested. When explaining tooth-brushing techniques to patients, the dental hygienist will demonstrate the method first then have the patient demonstrate the same technique. This is known as the "show-and-do" method. It focuses more on the participant than the teacher. It allows the educator to continue the demonstration while the learner follows along. Depending on the type of learning environment for a dental health presentation, the educator may also want to incorporate this interactive method.

As discussed, there are numerous ways to teach and learn. Anyone providing education has the opportunity to use multiple messages to enhance their presentation, which then allows the learner to absorb the information in a multitude of ways. All learning styles can be incorporated in the presentation so that whether an auditory or visual learner, the presentation addresses both.

Effective Communication

Interpersonal skills are essential to communication in any situation, whether it be with one patient or among a lecture hall of colleagues. Communication requires confidence in the topic being discussed or presented. Dental hygienists are well educated in oral health prevention, thus confident in recommendations made to patients as well as other arenas for dental health education. Communication has two sides: speaking and listening. It also includes allowing others to communicate their ideas. What is required to be an effective communicator?

First, it's best to identify how communication currently takes place: a self-evaluation. Figure 4.2 shows a list of questions designed to identify one's style. By identifying some of the things one may be doing now, changes can be made to improve one's style in the future. For example, if you are a part of a group of people you do not know and are huddled in one area of a conference room, are you participating in the conversation or are you only listening to the others? This may indicate lack of confidence either with the subject of the conversation or with people unknown to you. So how can changes be implemented? Perhaps, asking questions if the subject matter is unfamiliar. Or perhaps, being the first one to introduce yourself, and providing some background information on why you are attending the conference. This helps to break the ice, yet taking a lead in the exchange of conversation adds to confidence levels.

No matter how one answers these questions, information is gathered and can be incorporated in changing a current communication style that is ineffective to a style that is more effective. For example, if the speaker or communicator does not make a habit of remembering the names of others, it may send the message that those individuals are unimportant. If uncomfortable initiating a conversation, many will use the weather or sports as small talk. Small talk tends to allow people to warm up to more extensive conversation material.

---

1. When conversing with others, who does most of the talking?
2. When first meeting someone, who introduces themselves first?
3. Do I avoid small talk? Starting conversations?
4. Do I remember the names of others?
5. During a conversation, do I smile enough? Too much? Not at all?
6. Do I make eye contact? Sometimes? Not at all?
7. How is my body language? Am I standing too close? Sitting down while the other person is standing? Are my arms crossed?
8. Do others distract me? Do I allow myself to be interrupted by others?
9. Do I focus on negatives versus positives? Do I lead with negative comments?
10. Do I disagree without judgment? Does everyone have to see it my way?

FIGURE 4.2   Self-assessment questions for identifying communication styles. (Adapted from Jacobs, 2004)

Another example: How often does the dental hygienist focus on the negative versus the positive? Practitioners want their patients to have improved oral health and continue with the improvement at all times, yet when the 6-month follow-up visit comes around, does he or she comment on how great compliance is going? Or does the patient hear, "Well, it looks like there is some bacteria causing more inflammation in this area." What about all the other areas? Taking a step back to evaluate one's current communication style will be advantageous for the professional and those served by oral health education.

So now that identification of a current communication style has taken place, how can one build communication skills? Any skill acquired takes practice. Upon entering dental hygiene school, students realize how much practice it will take to learn the correct use of instruments. The same principle is applied with communication skills. Practicing new techniques will assist in making the process smooth and getting the message sent more effectively. By using some of the information from Figure 4.2, let's list some ways to overcome what may have been positive responses to the self-assessment questions.

Question 1: *When conversing with others, who does most of the talking?*

If engaged in a conversation, it is best to have equal parts in the dialogue. If one person does all the talking, is it a conversation? Probably not, it may be described more accurately as a lecture. So if you are the person doing all the talking, your exercise might be to be more aware of how little the other person is speaking, and allow them to initiate discussion and new subject matter.

When the dental hygienist asks their patients questions in order to obtain specific information, he or she will do well by allowing complete answers. Then repeating or providing feedback to clarify the answers being provided, the practitioner can be assured of information that may not have been brought out if he or she did all of the talking.

Question 7: *How is my body language? Am I standing too close? Sitting while the other person is standing? Are my arms crossed?*

Body language can say a lot about whether or not a person is open to conversation or accepting of others. If a patient is seated in the dental chair and the practitioner has asked a question, is the practitioner making eye contact or are they perhaps turned away looking at the patient chart? What this behavior indicates to the consumer is that the clinician is uninterested in the response, or may not even be listening to the response. One can improve this deficit in their communication style by paying attention and waiting until the patient has completed their response.

Distance between two people is another aspect to be aware of when working with patients. Everyone has his or her own "personal" space. When that space is invaded, a feeling of uneasiness occurs. For example, as a dental hygienist, face-to-face distance during debridement procedures may be at least 18 inches. When the clinician gets too close, the patient can feel invaded and uncomfortable. Allowing a comfortable space between the individuals engaged in conversation is something to work on for improving communication skills.

Eye contact is essential in communication, thus when in a discussion with a person standing or sitting, eye contact does not occur. There may also be a sense of inferiority in the person sitting. To alleviate this situation, the exercise would be to sit or stand as the person to whom you may be speaking.

Finally, if during a conversation one finds their arms are crossed in front of their body, the general message being sent may be that of defensiveness or being closed off. Finding a way to stand or sit comfortably with arms at your side or relaxed on your lap will indicate a more open and accepting attitude for conversation and communication.

As discussed, there are many things that can be done to initiate improved skills in communication.

1. Recognize and acknowledge the behaviors currently in place.
2. List ways to change or eliminate those behaviors.
3. Practice them during each and every communication opportunity.

Becoming an effective communicator will take time, yet by performing a self-assessment and identifying how to make appropriate changes, communication skills will begin to build quickly.

Summary

When communicating important information to an audience, it will be essential that the educator, whether a teacher or a dental professional, pays attention to the different learning styles of their audience. Self-assessment of one's own conversational style will assist in identifying where changes can occur so that anyone in conversation has equal and significant time. The skill of listening plays a key role in understanding what is being heard. Patients need to understand that the practitioner cares about them and are paying attention to their concerns. Understanding that there are those who learn well by auditory methods or visual methods will enhance the educator's style of presenting information. Handouts and lectures can incorporate numerous ways to address both learning styles and ensure that the audience can retain the information. The learning environment can either help or hurt the educator's presentation. Be prepared to change presentation styles based on the environment. Keep the audience interested in the topic by incorporating different methods of teaching such as small-group or interactive discussions.

To gain success at teaching dental education, prepare well by using multiple methods given the type of lesson being designed and the environment in which it is learned.

Critical Thinking

1. Explain the difference between listening and active listening.
2. List three areas from Figure 4.2 that you can identify for change or improvement in your current communication style.
3. Identify whether you are an auditory or visual learner. Describe the teaching methods that work more effectively for your learning process.

4. Explain the benefits of visual aids when discussing dental health with patients. How could you accomplish the same task without visual aids?

5. Describe the better learning environment for you and why it works. For example, do you require absolute silence? Do you need music or a television in the background?

Activities

1. Break into small groups and design an effective handout for a dental health topic.

2. Select a partner and practice active listening techniques.

3. Select a group of three students and have them begin a conversation. Using Figure 4-2, can the audience identify communication styles in each of the group members?

4. As a class, identify teaching learning methods that may enhance your learning. Incorporate these methods for one week with your instructor's assistance and compare the effectiveness to the previous method.

5. Using a video recorder, break into groups of two or three. Select an oral health topic and record the conversation for 2 minutes. View the recording and critique communication/listening styles.

References

Audrieth, A. L. "The Art of Using Humor in Public Speaking." http://www.squaresail.cin/auh.html, 1998.

Bull, K. S. "Creating Handouts to Accompany Presentations and Posters." Unpublished paper, Oklahoma State University, 2003.

Jacobs, R. "Building Effective Interpersonal Skills: Self Assessment Exercise." Unpublished paper, Portland Community College, 2004.

Robledo, S. J. *The Visual Learner.* http://www.parentcenter.com, 2004.

5

Learning Styles and Levels, Perceptions, and Trends—Part I: Prenatal to Adolescent

Objectives

Upon completion of this chapter, you will be able to

1. Educate the pregnant patient on the relationship between periodontal disease and preterm low birth weight babies.
2. Communicate effective techniques for implementation by expectant parents to reduce the risk of oral disease transmission to the newborn.
3. Apply an understanding of preschool-age learning styles in dental hygiene care and patient education.
4. Apply an understanding of early elementary–age learning styles in dental hygiene care and patient education.
5. Apply an understanding of middle school–age learning styles in dental hygiene care and patient education.

Introduction

Patients all have different ways in which they assimilate and utilize information, that is, different learning styles. It is vital that the dental hygienist recognize at an early stage in the clinician-to-patient relationship which comprehension and learning modalities best fit the individual. To accomplish this, the dental hygienist must consider many issues, including the stage of life of the patient, their socioeconomic status, and cultural influences. In

52

this chapter and the next, we examine these areas and how they vary throughout the stages of life.

Prenatal

As previously discussed in Chapter 3, the dental hygienist has an opportunity to affect not only the health of the pregnant patient, but also that of her child. There are several critical oral and total health topics that the pregnant woman should be made aware of, and the dental hygienist may be the only source of information on these topics for the patient. Unfortunately, oral health is often overlooked by medical professionals and consumers as part of prenatal medical care.

Whether a teen, adult, or older adult, the pregnant woman can be encouraged to enjoy her pregnancy as much as possible. It is an exciting time, often the healthiest time of a woman's life. Dental hygienists have important information to share with these patients that can be conveyed in a positive rather than a frightening manner.

The pregnant patient is often more focused on health than at any other time in her life. She becomes cognizant of the effect of her health and behaviors on the unborn baby. Hopefully, all are aware of the harmful effects of tobacco and alcohol use during pregnancy, and have committed to stop using these products. They should also be aware of the potential of damage to the baby due to drug use and may finally find the inspiration to stop this behavior as well. Caring for an unborn baby can be a powerful motivation for putting a stop to negative habits and developing positive ones.

The developing human fetus is vulnerable to harm from the effects of tobacco use by the expectant mother. There is a well-established correlation between cigarette smoking and preterm, low birth weight babies **(PLBW),** placenta previa, miscarriage, stillbirth, perinatal death, and sudden infant death syndrome (CDC, 2001). These and other harmful effects of tobacco use are well known, yet many Americans, including pregnant women, continue to smoke. (See Figure 5.1). Cigarette packaging even includes warnings about the risks of tobacco use to the unborn child.

The first trimester of pregnancy is when the organ systems of the embryo are forming. They are most susceptible to the harmful effects of tobacco during this period, although the other damaging effects will continue to manifest if smoking is continued throughout the pregnancy. The lips and palate are formed during the fourth and twelfth weeks, and are at an increased risk of developing with clefts with the mother's use of tobacco. The tooth buds may also be affected, resulting in delayed eruption.

Alcohol use during pregnancy puts the unborn baby at risk of **fetal alcohol syndrome (FAS),** which manifests with pre- and postnatal growth deficiencies; central nervous system anomalies, including mental, motor and learning disabilities; and facial dysmorphologies such as micrognathia, irregular ear shape and position, epicanthal eye folds, flattened midface, and an undersized nose with a reduced bridge height (National Center for Birth Defects and Developmental Disabilities, 2004).

As with tobacco use, the fetus is most susceptible to the harmful effects of alcohol use by the mother in the first trimester. The continued use of alcohol by the mother throughout pregnancy will increase the risks of spontaneous abortion and stillbirths. Heavy alcohol

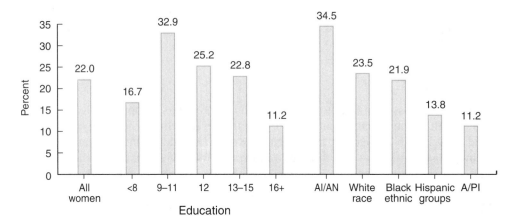

FIGURE 5.1 Prevalence of current smoking among women aged 18 years or older, all women, by education (1998), and by race/ethnicity (1997–1998), United States. (*Source:* National Health Interview Survey, 1997–1998)

use is not required for these harmful effects to occur; even occasional alcohol use during pregnancy has been shown to have damaging effects. Alcohol crosses the placental barrier easily, leaving the fetus vulnerable to mother's imbibing. And also, as with tobacco use, many women of childbearing age consume alcohol (Morbidity and Morbidity Weekly Report, 1994). Equipped with this knowledge and information, the dental hygienist is capable of educating a woman of childbearing age or pregnant patient of the consequences of alcohol consumption during pregnancy.

The use of elicit drugs such as cocaine, methamphetamines, and heroin is also harmful to the fetus. Possible outcomes include preterm low birth weight babies, microcephaly, postnatal seizures, and withdrawal symptoms (Wilkins, 1999). The patient may not be forthcoming with information of their ongoing use. The dental hygienist must be alert to signs and symptoms of drug abuse, including needle marks, altered pupil size, lack of interest in appearance, intoxicated behavior, neglected oral hygiene, and rampant caries.

If drug abuse is suspected, the dental hygienist will want to communicate concern and compassion. A defensive and resistant response is nearly inevitable when the patient is confronted with a "you should know better than that" attitude. The individual must be informed of the possible risks to the unborn baby. If the patient expresses a desire to quit, the dental hygienist can be prepared to assist with encouragement and possible referrals to professionals and organizations that are well versed in current cessation modalities.

Similarly, the pregnant patient that is using tobacco and/or alcohol should be informed of the possible outcomes with continued use. The need for communicating compassion is especially great when caring for a pregnant patient that is involved in these high-risk behaviors. Effecting positive changes will be more likely with encouragement and caring advice rather than with scolding. Specific guidelines for tobacco cessation in the nonpregnant patient will be discussed in a later chapter.

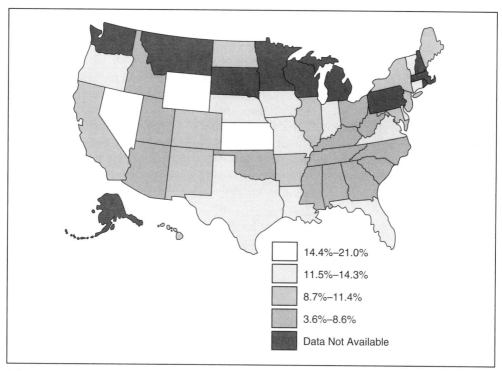

14.4%–21.0%

11.5%–14.3%

8.7%–11.4%

3.6%–8.6%

Data Not Available

* Consumed >30 drinks during the preceding month or ≥5 drinks on at least one occasion during the past month.

FIGURE 5.2   Percentage of frequent drinkers* among women of childbearing age, by quartile—Behavioral Risk Factor Surveillance System, 1991. (*Source:* Morbidity and Mortality Weekly Report, 1994)

Gingivitis occurs during many pregnancies. It occurs at such a frequent rate that many perceive it as "normal," but it has the potential to cause permanent harm to the periodontal tissues of the mother as well as contributing to the occurrence of PLBW babies (Darby & Walsh, 2003). The gingival and/or periodontal infection is not caused by pregnancy, but may be exacerbated by it. Hormonal changes can alter the tissue's response to bacterial plaque. The patient may not have experienced bleeding gingiva before the pregnancy even though she wasn't flossing regularly. It is often the case that the patient experiences bleeding when brushing or flossing during pregnancy, even though the amount of plaque is similar to prepregnancy levels.

When the pregnant patient understands that gingival bleeding during pregnancy is common yet still a pathology, and that there is a risk to the unborn baby if allowed to continue, motivation to improve oral hygiene habits is a natural outcome. The dental hygienist can encourage a pregnant patient to be more effective in plaque removal efforts in order to help slow or stop the progression of the gingival/periodontal infection. Effective daily flossing and twice-daily brushing should improve most "pregnancy gingivitis" situations. The dental hygienist should evaluate and monitor the periodontal condition of the pregnant woman and make appropriate recommendations if further treatment or more frequent dental hygiene care is indicated.

Regular brushing and flossing will also help to reduce the oral bacteria that will be passed on to the infant after delivery. Dental caries is an infectious disease. Babies are not born with the cariogenic pathogens. *Streptococcus mutans*, the main bacteria responsible for caries production, is often transferred by the parent to the child through the natural act of kissing the baby (Slavkin, 1997). Practitioners don't want to suggest that moms and dads stop kissing their babies, but encourage parents-to-be to begin oral care practices that will help prevent the transmission of these caries-causing bacteria, which are the following steps:

1. Parents should be examined and treated for any active carious lesions before the birth of the child.
2. Parents should be taught to effectively remove plaque from their oral surfaces by brushing and flossing daily.
3. Parents should consider using an antimicrobial dentifrice and mouthrinse to reduce their transmissible bacterial flora.

The expectant parent is usually receptive to information about preventing dental disease in their infant. The routine dental hygiene visit before the birth of the baby may be a prime opportunity to provide this instruction. Parents can be instructed to care for their infant's mouth even before the teeth begin to erupt:

1. The dental hygienist will want to be aware of the fluoride content of the community water supply and advise the parent of the need, if any, for supplementation.
2. The parent can be instructed to wipe the infant's mouth with a clean, damp cloth after feeding.
3. When the infant's teeth begin to erupt, they can be brushed gently by the parent with a damp, extra soft toothbrush without toothpaste.
4. Parents can be informed of the risk of **early childhood caries (ECC),** also known as *baby bottle syndrome* or *nursing bottle syndrome*, a rampant caries condition that is caused by improper feeding practices. Allowing liquids containing fermentable carbohydrates such as breast milk, formula, or juice to pool on the teeth, such as with a propped bottle, promotes ECC. Babies should not be put to bed with a bottle unless it contains water only.

Teen mothers are an especially at-risk group during pregnancy. Their pregnancies are often unplanned and unexpected. They may not seek prenatal care until the pregnancy is too obvious to ignore. The dental hygienist may be one of the first health care providers to make contact with the young pregnant woman and should be ready to provide information for her and her baby's health and dental health. The dental hygienist may recommend that she seek prenatal care as soon as possible if she hasn't already. She can also be encouraged to take particular care with her diet, supplementing with prenatal vitamins. Some teens have especially high nutritional demands during their pregnancies, particularly if they haven't finished growing themselves.

Preschool Age

Preschoolers, ages 2–5, are a fun but sometimes challenging age group to work with in the dental office. Their first dental office visit needs to be a pleasant experience, and some efforts may be made by the dental office staff and the dental hygienist in particular to make that possible. Understanding the learning levels of the child in this age group is part of that effort.

The preschool-age child is like a sponge, soaking up new information all the time from every possible source. Dental hygienists can be a source of the "good kind" of dental information that may pave the way for a pleasant dental office experience each time the child goes to the dentist for the rest of his or her life.

Preschoolers are sensory learners. They respond well to being able to explore and discover new places or ideas using as many of their senses as possible. Some dental offices encourage parents to bring little ones with them to their routine dental hygiene visits. This is a great opportunity for the toddler to become familiar with the office surroundings, equipment, and staff. The child can *hear* how the handpiece motor and the saliva ejector sounds. He can *see* the bright light the dental hygienist uses to see Mom or Dad's teeth. She can *feel* the rubber prophy cup with her fingers. He can *smell* the prophy paste or fluoride. The practitioner may want to leave *taste* out of this first experiential visit. A ride in the patient chair and having the preshooler's teeth "counted" may make this future patient really excited about being big enough to come to the dental office for his or her own visit.

Preschoolers are not usually physically able to adequately remove plaque from their teeth by themselves. Parents need to be educated on how to brush and floss the child's teeth regularly. It is important for oral care to be established as part of the daily routine, as much as combing hair or washing hands. Bath time is often a good time for the parent to take care of the child's brushing and flossing. To prepare the child for taking care of their own teeth, it is recommended to have the child brush after Mom or Dad, to "get what I might have missed." To reverse this process and have the parent brush after the child may send the message that "you can't do it well enough."

The parent should be instructed to use a pea-sized dab of toothpaste when brushing the child's teeth. Ingesting more than that amount of fluoride toothpaste on a regular basis will provide more fluoride than the child needs and may result in mild dental fluorosis in the permanent teeth. Some toddlers find toothpaste to be "too hot" and may resist brushing for this reason. The parent can try different toothpaste flavors until a flavor is discovered that is not objectionable to the child. This is actually more important than it may seem at first, but if the child doesn't like the toothpaste, chances are they won't brush their teeth long enough or adequately.

Elementary School Age

The elementary school–age child, around 6 to 11 years old, is able to process information and evaluate situations. Swiss psychologist Jean Piaget referred to this as the **concrete operations stage** (Dacey & Travers, 1999). These children will still respond well to having the equipment demonstrated and having questions answered. They will begin to understand the value of their oral health. They may have had friends that "got a shot in their mouth" or had an extraction, and that may contribute to a new fear of the dental office. This is an opportunity to provide correct information and guide the child into understanding the concept of preventing dental disease. The child needs to understand that the dentist and dental hygienist are a team; all three have *jobs* to do to prevent dental disease.

The *child's job* is to choose healthy snacks and brush their teeth well twice each day, especially at bedtime. Some children are able to floss their own teeth; others will need the parent to floss for them until their dexterity is more developed. The *dentist's job* is to examine the child's teeth twice yearly, looking for caries and orthodontic concerns. The dentist knows that it is best to discover dental problems before the patient perceives them. The treatment will usually be less involved, and therefore less uncomfortable or costly. The *dental hygienist's job* is to clean the child's teeth twice a year, removing accumulations of plaque, calculus, and stain. Fluoride applications are part of that cleaning and the child needs to understand the value of that fluoride treatment. Understanding the benefits of a topical fluoride application will help the school-age patient participate more willingly in the procedure. The dental hygienist is also checking for caries and orthodontic concerns as well as gingivitis. The dental hygienist provides oral hygiene instruction and/or correction as needed, and encouragement about dentally healthy snacks.

Middle School and Teen Age

The middle school–age and teenage child, around ages 12 to 18, has begun to look at the world around him with a more critical eye than the elementary school child. Presented with a statement of fact, an adolescent will often ask why or why not. While this may be a bit disconcerting to an adult that has infrequent contact with a young teen, questioning is a genuine attempt to gain a better understanding of the world around him. Understanding how and why things work is part of becoming an adult capable of making informed decisions.

Adolescents want and need to participate in their oral health care. This is the age that they need to take more responsibility for their teeth. They certainly don't want Mom or Dad to oversee their brushing and flossing anymore! They usually resent even being reminded to brush. These patients need to be made aware of dental diseases, including caries and gingivitis, and their role in exacerbating or preventing these diseases.

The dental hygienist is also charged with finding an individual reason for that patient to care. Most may remember thinking, *"That'll never happen to me."* Telling an adolescent that they must take better care of their teeth and gums or *someday* they may lose them may not be effective. *Someday* is for older people like their parents. Teenage patients need a reason to care *today* about what the dental hygienist has to say. Dental hygienists need to find a way to capture the teen's interest. When the dental hygienist finds a motivating factor, "hot button", the adolescent will be ready to learn.

There are several areas of adolescent interest that may be explored in order to find motivation for learning positive oral health practices. As discussed in the chapter on nutrition, it is helpful to learn what interests the individual teen patient. An athletic teen is probably interested in health and wellness for peak performance. The dental hygienist can explain the relationship between gingival/periodontal diseases and systemic disorders. A brief description of the bacteremia that occurs every time the patient experiences gingival bleeding may grab the teen's attention and interest. A good student with interest in scholastic pursuits may relate to the wisdom of choosing to develop good oral hygiene practices. A teen that is beginning to become interested in dating may respond to being shown photos or charts of attractive, healthy gingiva as opposed to "gross" pictures of gingival infection. Most teens are interested in fresh breath and often pop in a piece of gum for freshening. A description and demonstration of the odiferous bacterial compounds found in the interdental spaces and on the tongue may prove very motivating.

Summary

Several factors must be considered when developing an appropriate oral hygiene care recommendation for the dental patient: the stage of life, socioeconomic status, and individual values. In order to be an effective provider of vital information to the patient, the dental hygienist must weigh all of these. Humans learn throughout the lifespan in different styles and at different levels. Some areas of commonality may be identified for each stage.

Prenatal education involves two people at the same time. It is a special opportunity to influence the oral and total health of both the pregnant mother and her unborn baby. The dental hygienist is charged with providing information about behaviors that may harm the baby, the link between periodontal disease and PLBW, nutritional needs, how to reduce the risk of transferring oral pathogens to the newborn, and how to care for the newborn's oral tissues and eventually teeth. Expectant parents are typically nurturing and are receptive to oral health education from dental care professionals.

Preschool-age children are forming their lifelong dental perceptions with their first dental visits. The dental hygienist has the opportunity to make the first visit a positive experience by understanding that the preschooler is a sensory learner that needs to be allowed to physically discover (with guidance and supervision) the dental office. The child should not be expected to perform adequate plaque removal on his or her own, but can be guided into self-care by brushing after the parent.

Elementary school–age children need to understand more about the "why" part of how we do things. Explaining and teaching the child about oral disease, how it is caused, how it is prevented, and their role in that prevention will be more effective than simply telling the child what to do and how.

Middle school–age and teenage students are a tougher audience. When allowed to participate in informed choices about their oral health, most teens will choose positive oral health behaviors. It is especially helpful to find a "hot button" that will peak the patient's interest and provide the motivation needed to learn and implement these positive behaviors.

Critical Thinking

1. What can expectant parents do to reduce the risk of their child developing oral disease?
2. Briefly discuss the risks to the mother and unborn baby when the expectant mother develops gingivitis or periodontal disease.
3. How do preschoolers learn? How can this learning style be incorporated into the first dental visit?

Activities

1. Consider the following case: Kyle is 14 years old. His mother wanted him to be seen by the dental hygienist before beginning his orthodontic care. He is polite but very quiet. You have the impression that his mom's attention and yours embarrass him. His oral exam reveals heavy plaque and generalized acute gingivitis. Develop a dialogue that would engage Kyle into active interest and participation.
2. Your 8-year-old patient, Susan, is clearly anxious about her first visit to the dental office. She has been introduced to the dentist, and now you are conducting the initial exam. You discover rampant caries and an apical swelling above #3. What are your next steps?

References

Centers for Disease Control, National Center for Chronic Disease Prevention and Health Promotion. *Women and Smoking: A Report of the Surgeon General—2001.* http://www.cdc.gov/tobacco/sgr.

Dacey, J. S., and J. F. Travers. *Human Development across the Lifespan*, 4th ed. Boston: McGraw-Hill, 1999.

Darby, M. L., and M. M. Walsh. *Dental Hygiene Theory and Practice*, 2nd ed. Philadelphia: W. B. Saunders, 2003.

Morbidity and Mortality Weekly Report. *Frequent Alcohol Consumption among Women of Childbearing Age—Behavioral Risk Factor Surveillance System, 1991.* http://www.cdc.gov/epo/mmwr, 1994, May 13.

National Center for Birth Defects and Developmental Disabilities. *Fetal Alcohol Syndrome.* http://www.cdc.gov/ncbddd.fas, 2004.

Slavkin, H. C. First Encounters: Transmission of Infectious Oral Diseases from Mother to Child. *Journal of the American Dental Association, 128* (1997), 773–778.

Wilkins, E. M. *Clinical Practice of the Dental Hygienist*, 8th ed. Philadelphia: Lippincott, Williams & Wilkins, 1999.

6

Learning Styles and Levels, Perceptions and Trends—Part II: Adult to Elderly

Objectives

Upon completion of this chapter, you will be able to

1. Develop a personalized oral hygiene plan that incorporates the patient's needs, limitations, and abilities.
2. Recognize the factors to be considered when developing interventions for restoration or maintenance of oral health.
3. Recognize the behaviors or signs of the fearful patient and address the issues contributing to the fear.
4. Incorporate understanding and respect when developing a personalized oral hygiene plan for older patients.
5. Recognize the oral conditions that may be found with older patients.

Adulthood

Adults bring a complex mix of attitudes, experience, and values to the dental chair, all of which must be considered when developing a personalized oral hygiene education plan. There is not a "one-size-fits-all" approach available when it comes to adult oral health education. It must be individualized, based on each adult patient's dental condition, "**Dental I Q,**" values, socioeconomic status, education, and attitude. There is an unfortunate stereotypical perception of the dental hygienist as a caregiver that scolds about brushing and flossing every time he or she gets a patient in the chair. Let's face it, most adults will not accept being scolded or told what to do. The dental hygienist is therefore charged with finding an effective way to motivate and communicate with each patient that will provide the maximum opportunity for imparting valuable information.

The dental hygienist must have a clear goal or objective before developing the appropriate oral hygiene self-care plan for the patient. It is imperative that this goal is clearly stated to that patient. For example, during the initial assessment of patient Mary Smith's oral care needs, the dental hygienist observes several interproximal areas that bleed when probed. A goal may be "no bleeding on probing" by eliminating the causes of the inflammation that are causing the bleeding. Part of that elimination process is the dental hygiene instrumentation. Another important aspect is the daily plaque removal by Mrs. Smith, in this case, with dental floss. She will be informed of her condition (periodontal disease, gingivitis), what caused it, the goal of health and what the interventions of the dental hygienist will be to assist in achieving that goal.

Using the condition of Mrs. Smith described above, let's explore the factors that must be considered before presenting the information to the patient:

1. **Dental condition.** Mary Smith has localized gingivitis in some interproximal areas. There doesn't appear to be a problem with the patient's brushing, but Mary is not flossing regularly (usually only when food is caught).

2. **"Dental I Q."** This is a reference to the patient's existing knowledge or awareness of their condition, the treatment options, and prevention of disease. This is not a judgment of their overall intelligence as highly educated, intelligent persons may be unaware of their oral condition or the consequences of oral disease. Some patients aren't interested in treatment until they have experienced pain. Mrs. Smith had noticed occasional bleeding but thought it was "normal."

3. **Values.** Does this patient value his or her teeth? Is there an expectation of keeping these teeth for a lifetime? Or are dentures an acceptable option? Is an attractive smile important to this individual? How about fresh breath? Is the ability to powerfully crunch down on the hardest carrot important? Dental hygienists need to be aware that not all people think teeth are that important. The dental hygienist may discover that the first task in this patient's oral hygiene education is to help the individual learn to value their teeth. Mary says that she desires a nice smile and fresh breath, an indication that she places some value in healthy teeth and gingiva.

4. **Socioeconomic status.** The cost of a dental appointment is an important consideration to many patients. Employees may or may not have a dental plan in their benefits package. Retirees often choose not to pick up the option of dental insurance with their medical plan due to a reduction in their incomes. Dental hygienists must consider that their recommendation for dental office continuing care (maintenance) may not be followed if the patient has fixed-income considerations. The dental hygienist will need to describe the economic sense of preventive care. Mary has a new job that offers dental insurance as a benefit, so for the first time in many years she feels like she can afford regular dental care "as long as the insurance pays for it."

5. **Education.** Patients come to our dental offices with varying levels of education. An individual with a degree in biological science may need an explanation of the dental disease process that is more comprehensive and science-based than most. The patient with less formal education still needs a description of their disease process, but perhaps in terminology more appropriate for that individual. Mary is an elementary school teacher. She expresses an interest in learning about why and how to achieve and maintain optimal oral health.

6. **Attitude.** Does the patient seem interested in the dental hygienist's information? Is he or she here only because their spouse made the appointment? Does the clinician notice that the patient is frequently glancing at the clock? The individual may seem distracted or uninterested at this particular appointment because of something that is going on with him or her on this particular day. This may not be the best day for an in-depth revamping of their oral hygiene routine. When the dental hygienist perceives that this is the case, notations can be made in the patient's chart. Future visits may prove more mutually productive. The patient, Mary Smith, is busy and involved yet her attitude conveys interest and respect.

The Fearful Adult

An unfortunate reality of dentistry is that many people are fearful of the dental office visit. A fearful dental patient will present with a variety of responses and behaviors that may interfere with the provision of dental care.

The most common expression of the fearful dental patient is that they don't come in to the office. They tend to not schedule preventive or elective dental care appointments. A toothache is hard to ignore, so dental emergency appointments may be the only appointments that are scheduled. Another coping mechanism may be to schedule the appointment but fail to keep it. The individual may call to cancel and not reschedule or they may just not show.

If a fearful patient does manage to make it into the dental hygienist's chair, they may present with a variety of signs and symptoms that may alert the clinician of their anxiety. The most common signs include:

- elevated blood pressure and pulse
- increased perspiration (especially upper lip, brow, and palms)
- xerostomia
- talking too much or too loud
- not talking
- wiggling or fidgeting
- white knuckles
- unfriendly, sullen demeanor

When these signs and symptoms are recognized by the dental hygienist, action must be taken to alleviate the fear or anxiety. Communication is the first step and the most important one. The clinician needs to convey understanding, empathy, and reassurance to the patient.

Dentistry has come a long way in the past three decades or so. Pain management is now an expectation of dental care, but it wasn't always so. Many adult patients recall being scolded by the dental staff when they were children if they cried because the caries evacuation (drilling) was painful. Or they may recall being deprived of a toy because they weren't "good" for the dentist. Most dental care personnel have had at least one patient tell them about the horrible extraction they had where they weren't numb and the doctor had to put his foot on the patient's chest to "yank" out the tooth! This is a highly doubtful scenario, but like an urban legend, the story seems to continue.

The media depiction of dentistry isn't helpful either. Some portrayals are intended as humorous, and they truly are funny for the dentally secure public. Bill Cosby performed a terrific portrayal as a patient that is having a carious lesion prepared for a restoration. Between being numb and the dentist never removing his hands from Bill's mouth, poor Mr. Cosby is helplessly unable to communicate his concerns. He thinks there's smoke coming out of his mouth. It's a delightful performance to watch. Tim Conway had a classic skit as the bumbling dentist that manages to get every part of his own anatomy anesthetized with an overly large syringe, but can't get it into the patient's mouth. Great fun! But for those with **dental anxieties** or phobias, these portrayals may contribute to their fears. One of the most frightening portrayals of dental torture is in a film that shows one of the main characters trying to elicit information from another by boring into a vital incisor without anesthetic.

If the origin of fear is known to the patient, the management by the dental professional is much easier. If the patient is able to tell the clinician about something that happened that was particularly unpleasant, the dental hygienist will be able to address that issue. If the last dental hygiene visit was so painful that the patient didn't want to come back, the dental hygienist will want to attempt to discover if the pain was during the procedure or after, and let the patient know that there are tools available to keep that from happening again. Empowerment is a powerful tool for the patient. The individual may be requested to tell the clinician or give a hand signal when something is painful. The dental hygienist may tell the patient that instrumentation will stop when given the signal. The clinician must be prepared to respond to these signals, otherwise the trust that was developing will evaporate.

Relaxation techniques are effective for some patients. Soothing music in the operatory or on the patient's own headset may be helpful. Pausing for deep breathing may help to calm both the patient and the clinician. Nitrous oxide sedation or an antianxiety premedication may be required for the most anxious patients.

The ability of dental hygienists in some states to administer local anesthesia during the course of dental hygiene care has helped many patients. This ability has allowed dental hygienists to become more involved in nonsurgical periodontal care as well. While not usually required for routine dental hygiene care, the fearful patient may be comforted to know that anesthesia is an option.

Pain control also includes correct instrumentation techniques. The patient's previous discomfort may have been due to an earlier clinician's use of heavy lateral pressure to compensate for a dull instrument. Another problem may be a curet that has been incorrectly sharpened to a point. Poor adaptation also causes unnecessary tissue trauma. Postoperative suggestions such as warm saline rinses and ibuprofen as needed are also helpful. Less postoperative pain will increase the likelihood of that patient returning for more dental hygiene care.

 # Older Adults

Aged patients represent even more diversity in background. They should not be categorized as a homogenous entity. Some older patients have retired, some are working because of need or desire, and some are physically challenged for the first time in their lives. It is helpful to anticipate some of the barriers that may be presented when providing oral health education to older adult patients. Dental hygienists will customize dental health education to fit the aged individual's needs and abilities. The following issues must not be considered to be typical of all older patients. Many have adjusted to their situations very well. Considering the possible challenges facing the aged patient will help the dental care professional to better understand and manage the dental care of these individuals.

 # Identity

Changing roles throughout the lifespan contribute to a change in perception of identity. When asked to tell about themselves, most people will state what they do, such as "I'm an accountant" or "I have three children." In later years, the children are grown and are no longer part of everyday "busyness." Retirement from many years of employment is the norm for older adults. Both of these scenarios represent major changes in self-perception. Abraham Maslow placed self-esteem and self-actualization at the top of his **hierarchy of human needs** (see Figure 6.1). Both may be challenged or lacking in older patients.

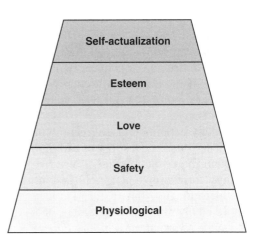

FIGURE 6.1 Abraham Maslow's hierarchy of human needs.

Healthy teeth and a nice smile may have been important to the older individual during the busy adult years. As a parent, the patient may have been motivated to demonstrate positive oral health practices as role models for their children. Working with the public may have been a powerful incentive for maintaining a healthy smile and fresh breath. When those roles have changed, the dental hygienist may discover that older patients may lose interest in their teeth, unless a problem develops. The dental hygienist may need to help stimulate a renewed interest in oral health.

Habits

One of the common obstacles to learning positive oral health practices is the aged patient's concept of "I've been doing it this way for years. It was all right for the last 65 years, why should I change now?" The problem is that many self-care efforts may have seemed "all right," but were actually not. Many years of brushing with a scrubbing motion, for example, may eventually result in gingival recession and abraded cementum. This brushing technique may not have been noticed by the dental care providers until the damage became evident.

When attempting to change an older patient's oral hygiene habits, it is common for the dental hygienist to be confronted with resistance. Some older individuals may even insist that they are too old to change. In order for the patient to change what they've been doing, they have to believe that it is worth changing. The dental hygienist must show the patient evidence of the damage and explain the consequences of not modifying the technique. It is important to respect and not criticize the aged patient. The individual can be encouraged to make the choice to change what they've been doing in order to preserve their dentition. Then, the corrections and suggestions can be made gradually and regularly at subsequent appointments.

Limited Income

Many older patients are on a "fixed" income, which may be an ongoing concern. Working people, even self-employed, have the expectation or hope of regular increases in their incomes. Retirement income is typically at a fixed rate that does not increase along with the cost of living. So when the cost of their semi-annual dental hygiene visit increases by a seemingly minor 10% over last year's price, the patient may express a degree of anxiety or frustration.

Many patients choose to come in for dental hygiene care once yearly instead of twice. They may also request fewer radiographs to cut down on costs. The dental hygienist must explain the possible risks of less frequent preventive care. Without the benefit of regular x-rays, for example, a carious lesion may go unnoticed until it has progressed to the pulp of the tooth. A simple restoration is no longer an option. Now the patient may need a much more costly root canal treatment or he or she may even lose the tooth. The dentist should be made aware of the patient's concerns and choices.

Physical Challenges

Some physical limitations may inhibit the aged patient's ability to care for his or her teeth. There may also be changes that need to be considered in order for the individual to receive care and for mutual communication to occur. (See also Chapter 7.)

1. **Hearing loss.** The patient may have reduced hearing ability. Signs of hearing loss include inappropriate or lack of response, frequently requesting the clinician to repeat what was said, or turning one side toward the clinician (hearing may be better in one ear than in the other).

   The dental hygienist can improve communication with the hearing impaired patient by reducing the ambient sounds, turning down music in the operatory if possible. Conversation with this individual should be conducted with the clinician facing the patient. The face mask should not be covering the clinician's mouth. Many hard-of-hearing people are aided in understanding conversations by seeing their lip movements. Speech needs to be clear and slow with volume increased gradually as indicated.

   Today's hearing aids are quite effective for many types of hearing impairment. If the patient is wearing a hearing aid, the clinician may not need to increase the volume of his or her voice; which may prove to be irritating to the individual. The hearing aid should be removed or turned off during instrumentation, especially if ultrasonic instrumentation is utilized.

2. **Visual impairment.** The dental hygienist should be aware that the patient may not be able to see visual aids or demonstrations without corrective lenses. If the individual's corrective lenses have been exchanged for safety glasses for the appointment, the clinician will need to give the glasses back to the patient for oral hygiene instruction demonstrations.

3. **Mobility impairment.** The aged patient may need assistance from the clinician while entering and exiting the dental operatory and chair. If the individual is using a walker or cane, the clinician will want to clear obstacles such as loose rugs, rheostats, hoses, and cords. The operatory chair should be raised or lowered to the height of the patient's knees before seating. After the individual is seated, the cane or walker is placed out of the way, but within the patient's line of sight and reach. Assisting the individual in this manner is a natural, caring thing to do. It will also help to establish the trust, confidence, and rapport that is so important in the patient–clinician relationship.

   Limited mobility will also be a factor in oral hygiene. The patient may not be able to grasp or manipulate the toothbrush or dental floss effectively due to arthritis or other conditions.

4. **Medical issues.** The health history is especially important when providing dental care to the aged patient. The interview should be conducted in a quiet, private setting and in a caring, unhurried manner. Each question should be presented separately rather than in a list, allowing the patient to consider each issue carefully. The clinician can anticipate that this portion of the appointment will take extra time. If the clinician is not feeling rushed and anxious, the patient will likely feel less anxious as well. This intimate

exchange is often the beginning of a rewarding, professional relationship between the clinician and the older individual. The findings discovered in the medical history interview may lead to modifications in the dental appointment. The dental hygienist may be the first to suggest the need for antibiotic premedication for a medical condition. The clinician may discover that one or more of the patient's medications have oral side effects. The clinician may also find that with a particular medication or condition the individual must be seated in a semi-supine position rather than fully supine. Again, the patient will likely appreciate the clinician's awareness and consideration of their health, which will contribute to their confidence and trust.

Oral Considerations

The oral findings will dictate the modifications that need to be communicated to the aged patient, as with all patients. As discussed earlier, there is no such thing as a blanket oral hygiene recommendation for older patients. The following are some of the oral conditions that may be found in older patients.

1. **Gingival recession.** Years of aggressive toothbrushing, using a hard-bristled toothbrush, periodontal disease, or occlusal stresses may leave the aged patient with several areas of gingival recession. Exposed cementum is less mineralized than enamel and therefore more vulnerable to attack from plaque acids. Root caries progresses more rapidly than caries involving enamel. The dental hygienist may recommend gentle but thorough cleansing of the entire tooth surface. Multiple fluoride exposures are recommended as well, in the form or toothpastes, rinses, and home fluoride gel applications.

2. **Xerostomia.** A dry mouth is common in older patients. The causes are many, and include radiation therapy, Sjögren's syndrome, and medications. When the dental hygienist reviews the patient's medical history, particular attention should be paid to the oral effects of medications. Many prescription medications may cause xerostomia. A dry mouth is uncomfortable, making chewing and swallowing difficult, and may put the individual at increased risk for caries, particularly root caries.

   The dental hygienist cannot recommend that the patient stop taking the medications that are contributing to the xerostomia. Rather, the dental hygienist will make recommendations that contribute to the individual's comfort and reduce the caries risk. These include frequent sips of water; use of a home humidifier; avoidance of hard candies, mints, or lozenges containing sugar; use of an oral rinse that moistens the tissues; avoidance of alcohol-containing mouthrinses; meticulous plaque removal; and the use of a fluoride. As with the patient with exposed cementum, fluoride may be in the patient's dentifrice, a mouthrinse, and a home-use gel.

3. **Plaque retention.** There are several factors that may contribute to the accumulation of plaque on the oral surfaces in the aged patient. Exposed cementum is not as smooth as enamel and is therefore more likely to retain plaque. Gingival recession and loss of alveolar bone may result in wide embrasures that will hold food debris and plaque.

Restorations and prostheses provide an increased surface area for plaque accumulation, as well as challenges with the individual's cleaning efforts.

Specific instructions may be demonstrated to help the patient with plaque removal efforts. The use of an interproximal brush and floss threaders will help with some of the difficult to maintain areas, but some individuals may have difficulty maneuvering these implements. Dexterity may be limited due to conditions such as arthritis or Parkinson's disease. It may be helpful to modify the handle of the toothbrush to make it easier to grasp. Patients that demonstrate an inability to effectively remove plaque with manual efforts may benefit from the use of a power toothbrush.

 # Nutritional Considerations

As discussed in Chapter 3, there are several possible nutritional issues that must be evaluated when developing the appropriate oral hygiene care plan for the aged patient. When the patient assessment reveals findings that may indicate excesses or deficiencies in nutrients, the dental hygienist may consider a nutritional assessment. Oral hygiene recommendations will be less effective than they should be, if for example, the individual's habit of sucking on hard candies most of the day has not been addressed.

Summary

Adult learners come with a wide mix of attitudes and experiences that must be respected. The patient's individual dental condition, overall existing knowledge of dental health and dental care, value systems (particularly their dental values), socioeconomic status, education, and attitude are quickly considered while the dental hygienist finds the best dental health education plan for them.

Fear of dental care may prevent the patient from receiving the dentistry they need. The dental hygienist is an integral part of restoring the individual's confidence in safe, comfortable dentistry through communication, compassion, and quality care.

Older adults are faced with even more diverse backgrounds than younger adults, simply due to their years of life experience. In addition to the previous considerations, the dental hygienist must also consider and respect their changing identities, long-standing habits, limited income, and physical challenges. The aged patient may also present with oral conditions such as recession, xerostomia, and plaque retention problems, which must be addressed. Nutritional considerations are important as well, and are considered in more detail in Chapter 3.

 # Critical Thinking

1. What are the factors that must be considered when developing an adult patient's oral hygiene recommendations?

2. What can a dental hygienist do to motivate an adult learner to implement positive oral health habits?

3. How can a dental hygienist help to develop trust and rapport when working with an older patient?

4. What recommendations should be made for the patient with xerostomia?

5. What are the signs and symptoms of the fearful dental patient?

Activities

1. Role play: One student is an 82-year-old patient with osteoarthritis. The patient receives regular dental hygiene care and is not aware of any problems with his or her teeth. The other student is the dental hygienist. The clinician has discovered xerostomia, six carious lesions on root surfaces, and heavy plaque. Conduct a possible dialogue that will communicate the dental hygienist's recommendations and the patient's possible limitations and frustrations.

2. Role play: One student is a 45-year-old patient, the other is the dental hygienist. The patient is in the dental chair because his or her spouse made the appointment. This individual has not received regular care in the past because it wasn't in the family budget, nothing hurts, and "it's almost time for dentures anyway." Now the spouse has a job with dental insurance. The individual brushes *almost* every day, has gingival bleeding with brushing ("Isn't that normal?"), and also notices an unpleasant breath odor. Develop a dialogue between the dental hygienist and the patient that will address the issues of this individual and how those issues may be managed by the clinician.

Reference

Dacey, John S. and John F. Travers, *Human Development Across the Lifespan* Fourth ed. Boston: McGraw Hill, 1999.

7

Special Needs Populations

Objectives

Upon completion of this chapter, the dental hygiene student will be able to

1. Describe the possible implications of lack of access to dental hygiene care.
2. Identify systemic diseases or conditions that contribute to oral disease.
3. Design an oral health care regimen for the medically compromised patient.
4. Identify features of the dental office and operatory that impede access to care.
5. Design and present adaptive oral hygiene instruction for the patient with physical, mental, or sensory impairments.

Introduction

As part of providing dental hygiene care, the dental hygienist needs to have a complete picture of the health of the individual patient. This picture includes not only physical health, but also mental and emotional health. Patients with limitations and challenges may present with oral health conditions and issues that are not seen in individuals without apparent limitations. Understanding these challenges will help to ensure that the dental hygienist is providing appropriate dental hygiene care.

In Esther M. Wilkins's *Clinical Practice of the Dental Hygienist* (2005), it becomes apparent that all dental hygiene patients are special and have unique needs. These needs are considered when developing the treatment plan and patient education. A patient with a high caries rate has special needs. An individual with financial challenges has special needs. An older person living alone has special needs. Wilkins also states that "the dental hygienist's obligation is to see that no patient needs special rehabilitative dental or periodontal services because of any condition that could have been prevented by dental hygiene care" (p. 650).

The American Dental Hygienists Association Code of Ethics states the basic belief that "all people should have access to healthcare, including oral healthcare." As part of the professional responsibility dental hygienists must "serve all clients without discrimination and avoid action toward any individual or group that may be interpreted as discriminatory." This chapter is intended to help the dental hygiene student recognize potential barriers to dental hygiene care, understand the physical and mental challenges faced by many, and develop individualized and appropriate oral health education for each patient.

The Challenges Faced by the Patient with Special Needs

Identifying the Patient with Special Needs

As previously stated, all patients are special. However, certain individuals may have conditions that require modifications by their health care providers in order to ensure provision of adequate and appropriate care. Careful review of the health history may reveal conditions that require treatment modification. For example, antibiotic prophylaxis is advised for the patient with a mitral valve prolapse. It is the dental hygienist's responsibility to make sure that the patient scheduled for dental hygiene care has taken the prescribed antibiotic at the appropriate time (usually one hour before the procedure). Another example may be the patient with mental retardation that may need assistance with personal hygiene. Additionally, the dental hygienist may need to determine whether to include the care provider when oral hygiene instruction is provided instead of or in conjunction with the patient.

Access to Dental Health Care

Everyone is entitled access to dental health care. Lack of dental insurance or other financial means is a barrier to many, as discussed in Chapter 2. In the not too distant past, a physical or mental challenge would also be a barrier to access to dental health care. In the 1950s, special needs persons were referred to as "shut-ins" because they were literally shut inside their homes or institutions. Public facilities such as schools, shopping areas, or entertainment venues were rarely designed to accommodate persons with physical limitations. Societal changes have provided the general public with a better understanding of the needs and rights of these individuals. (Later in this chapter, mandated regulations providing physical accessibility will be discussed.) In modern society, no patient should be without access to dental health care.

Consequences of Unmet Dental Health Needs

Any individual that rarely or never visits a dental office is at risk for oral disease. Preventive dental care is by definition designed to avoid unnecessary and sometimes painful dental disease. Periodic radiographs provide the dentist with the ability to diagnose early carious lesions before the patient is able to detect discomfort or sensitivity. Radiographs are also used by the dental hygienist in the determination of the patient's periodontal status. Removal of calculus deposits by the dental hygienist helps to eliminate a **nidus** for harmful bacteria that contribute to periodontal diseases. It is recommended that this procedure be performed regularly to help prevent periodontal diseases.

A person without access to regular dental care is not likely to be aware of a carious lesion until the lesion nears or invades the pulpal tissue of the tooth. The lesion that was recognizable in its early stages could have been treated with a small restoration. The lesion that has invaded the dental pulp compromises the vitality of the tooth. The restoration of that tooth may require extensive dental procedures including root canal therapy and possibly a crown. Left untreated, the tooth could possibly abscess, often painfully, necessitating immediate endodontic therapy or an extraction. Similarly, a person that is not able to receive regular dental hygiene care may continue to accumulate calculus on the tooth and root surfaces. This will not only provide an increase in the surface area for bacterial accumulation, but will also deny the possibility of early intervention (removal of dental deposits, oral hygiene instruction, chemotherapeutic utilization) by the dental hygienist that could arrest or eliminate the progression of periodontal disease.

Providing dental hygiene care to the special needs patient may be physically and/or mentally challenging for the dental hygienist and the patient. Focusing on the individual's abilities rather than disabilities will make the dental hygiene care process more positive for all involved, and consequences such as those previously mentioned can be avoided.

The Medically Compromised Patient

Heart Disorders

Several heart conditions play roles in the provision of dental hygiene care. The patient with rheumatic heart disease is at risk for **infective endocarditis (IE).** This is a serious condition that may result in more heart damage, congestive heart failure or cerebrovascular disease. Individuals with a history of rheumatic fever should be informed that they are susceptible to rheumatic heart disease, which may cause permanent damage to the heart valves as well as susceptibility to IE. To reduce this risk, the patient with a history of rheumatic heart disease will be recommended to consult a physician to determine the presence or absence of cardiac damage. The dental hygienist must educate the individual on the possibility of transient **bacteremia** (elevated levels of microorganisms in the blood) with dental hygiene care that may contribute to IE. The patient must also understand that transient bacteremia occurs with self-care procedures such as brushing and flossing whenever the individual experiences gingival bleeding.

Patients at risk of IE due to rheumatic heart disease, mitral valve prolapse with regurgitation, or prosthetic heart valves require antibiotic therapy **(prophylactic antibiotic premedication)** before invasive dental appointments. (See Table 7.1.) An individual at risk is more likely to take responsibility for following the necessary recommendations before dental care if educated on the possible consequences of invasive dental care without antibiotic premedication. Prophylactic antibiotic premedication prior to the patient performing

TABLE 7.1 American Heart Association Recommendations for Prophylactic Antibiotic Coverage for Select Dental Procedures for Individuals at Risk for Infective Endocarditis

Standard recommendation	Amoxicillin (oral)	Adult Child	2.0 g 1 hour before procedure 50 mg/kg 1 hour before procedure
Allergic to penicillin	Clindamycin (oral) or	Adult Child	600 mg 1 hour before procedure 20 mg/kg 1 hour before procedure
	Cephalexin or Cefadroxil (oral) or	Adult Child	2.0 g 1 hour before procedure 50 mg/kg 1 hour before procedure
	Azithromycin or Clarithromycin (oral)	Adult Child	500 mg 1 hour before procedure 15 mg/kg 1 hour before procedure
Unable to take oral medication	Ampicillin (IM or IV)	Adult Child	2.0 g within 30 minutes before procedure 50 mg/kg within 30 minutes before procedure
Allergic to penicillin and unable to take oral medication	Clindamycin (IV) or	Adult Child	600 mg within 30 minutes before procedure 20 mg/kg within 30 minutes before procedure
	Cefazolin (IM or IV)	Adult Child	1.0 g within 30 minutes before procedure 25 mg/kg within 30 minutes before procedure

self-care procedures is neither practical nor recommended. This individual with a thorough understanding of the effects of bacteremia may be more likely to perform adequate oral hygiene procedures to maintain gingival and periodontal health.

Individuals with **ischemic heart disease** are at risk for angina pectoris, congestive heart failure, and myocardial infarction. The ischemia is usually the result of atherosclerosis, where the arteries supplying the cardiac muscle become narrowed or occluded by fatty plaques. The dental hygienist will want to encourage and reinforce recommendations from the patient's cardiologist, such as compliance through medication, exercise, reductions in animal fat consumption, and not smoking.

Several cardiovascular diseases require the use of anticoagulant therapy to prevent the formation of blood clots and artery blockage. Warfarin (Coumadin) is an anticoagulant medication that is often used for patients with thrombophlebitis or at risk for a myocardial infarction. This therapy may result in prolonged bleeding after invasive dental care. The dental hygienist will want to consult with the patient's physician in advance of the dental hygiene appointment to determine the **prothrombin time.** The physician may recommend temporary reduction or cessation of the anticoagulant therapy.

Diabetes

The patient with diabetes is at increased risk for some oral diseases. Reduced salivary flow, elevated salivary glucose, and altered healing response in the individual with poorly controlled blood glucose levels increase the risk of caries and periodontal diseases. Complete dental hygiene care includes educating the patient of these risks. Similar to the education provided to the individual with cardiovascular disease, the dental hygienist will reinforce and encourage compliance with the recommendations of the physician. Some persons with diabetes are advised to self-test their blood glucose levels regularly, and should be encouraged to do so. The dental hygienist will also want to reinforce the nutrition, exercise, and medication recommendations of the physician.

Oral hygiene efforts of the patient with diabetes are particularly important. The increased oral disease risks must be communicated to the individual with diabetes. Regular fluoride exposures in dentifrices, oral rinses, and gels will help to reduce the risk of caries. Use of an antimicrobial mouthrinse may also be recommended. Plaque removal with a toothbrush and dental floss should be as effective as possible. The dental hygienist will evaluate the efficacy of these efforts at each dental hygiene care visit. Regular and effective plaque removal will also help to reduce the risk of gingival and periodontal infections in the patient with diabetes. (See Chapter 8.)

Cancer

The individual undergoing chemotherapy and/or radiation therapy for cancer will experience oral side effects that require management by the dental care team. Radiation therapy, particularly in the head and neck region, may result in xerostomia, mucositis, and rampant caries. Chemotherapy can contribute to immunosuppression, nausea and vomiting, anemia, and loss of appetite. Orally, chemotherapy can cause painful ulcerative mucositis, making nutrient intake more challenging (Palmer, 2003). The dental care team has opportunities and responsibilities to these individuals before, during, and after their cancer treatments.

When presented with the opportunity to provide dental hygiene care to the cancer patient before they begin treatment, the dental hygienist and dentist can work together to eliminate sources of potential infection, including recurrent caries, root tips, overhanging restoration margins, ill-fitting prostheses, and calculus accumulations. The dental professional can educate the patient regarding the immunosuppressive effects of chemotherapy and elective dental care may need to be postponed during the course of the cancer treatment. The oncologist may be consulted before dental care during chemotherapy, as the physician may recommend prophylactic antibiotic premedication. (See Table 7.1.) The dental hygienist can also educate about the potential oral effects of chemotherapy or radiation therapy. A home fluoride preparation can be provided before radiation therapy begins, with instructions to use it regularly before, during, and after treatment to protect the teeth and root surfaces from the effects of xerostomia (rampant caries).

Once radiation or chemotherapy has begun, the patient can focus on disease prevention, yet place extra emphasis on issues affecting comfort, nutrient intake, and prevention of injury. The mucous membranes and other oral tissues may be more easily damaged during cancer therapy, particularly chemotherapy, than at other times (Palmer, 2003).

Patients that routinely use interproximal brushes or picks may be advised to discontinue this practice until tissues have returned to normal. Super-soft-bristled toothbrushes are recommended in order to aid in the prevention of injury to the altered oral tissues. The brush should be regularly disinfected with **chlorhexidine gluconate,** and should be replaced frequently to help reduce potentially harmful microorganisms. Chlorhexidine rinses may also be recommended; however, the patient will want to be informed that it may cause temporary discomfort on inflamed oral tissues. Saline rinses may provide some soothing relief to tissues. Any over-the-counter mouthrinses that are recommended are best if they are alcohol-free due to the tissue condition during chemotherapy. Radiation therapy patients need to continue regular use of the fluoride preparation previously recommended. These individuals are also advised to eat soft, nutrient-dense foods that are not overly spicy.

After treatment for cancer, there may be personal considerations that can affect dental hygiene care. The treatments may have caused disfigurement, may not have been successful, may have strained the family budget, or there may be residual pain. It is helpful to understand some of these issues when providing dental hygiene care and patient education. These considerations often manifest into fear, anxiety, and unexpected behaviors, such as frequent appointment cancellation or mood changes during the course of the appointment. The focus of oral health education for these individuals may need to be more comfort-oriented now, versus on the prevention of future oral diseases.

Respiratory Disorders

Individuals with a respiratory system disorders such as asthma, **chronic obstructive pulmonary disease (COPD),** and tuberculosis are susceptible to oral effects of the diseases and/or their treatment. Dental health education provided by the clinician for these patients will include prevention of related oral conditions and encouragement and support of managing their total health.

The patient with asthma often requires the use of inhalers for delivery of their medications. These and other medications may have serious oral effects. Xerostomia is a possible side effect of some, candidiasis is another. Due to the unpleasant flavor of some inhalants, some persons with asthma, especially children, habitually consume candy or gum to combat the bad taste. The frequent sucrose exposure compounds the caries-contributing effects of xerostomia. The patient with asthma can be encouraged to rinse with water after using the inhaler to decrease the risk of caries and candidiasis. Sugar-free gum is also recommended, as it will improve the taste in the mouth, as well as stimulate salivary flow.

The two most common conditions of COPD are chronic bronchitis and emphysema. Both of these conditions may be caused by cigarette smoking, working around noxious materials, and exposure to air pollutants. Individuals who suffered from severe respiratory illness as children are also susceptible to COPD. In addition to inhaler use, these patients may be taking corticosteroids. The dental hygienist will want to consult with their physician who may recommend supplementing the corticosteroid dosage for dental appointments. Intermediate-range steroid dosage (20–40 mg/day hydrocortisone or 5–10 mg/day prednisone) may necessitate additional dosages if the dental procedure is likely to contribute to a severe stress response (Requa-Clark, 415). These patients can also be instructed in the prevention of oral diseases related to the use of inhalers.

Tuberculosis (TB) is a communicable bacterial disease that affects the lungs as well as other organs and tissues. In spite of the success in treatment of this disease with antibiotics, it remains one of the most prevalent diseases in the world (WHO, 2002). This is due to certain high-risk lifestyles or living conditions that may result in inadequate access to treatment or failure to complete treatment (CDC, 2003). The antibiotic course for the treatment of tuberculosis takes a minimum of 6 months. Patient compliance is mandatory for positive resolution. Failure to complete the antibiotic therapy has resulted in an upsurge of antibiotic-resistant tuberculosis microbes. The dental hygienist should assess the patient's understanding of the importance of completion of the antibiotic regime, and the individual is encouraged to comply. Consultation with the patient's physician will provide information on the current infectious status, as infectious patients with tuberculosis are likely not to be treated in usual clinical settings.

All patients that smoke, particularly those with respiratory diseases, should be encouraged in smoking cessation. Chapter 8 will address smoking cessation methodologies.

The Patient in a Long-Term Care Facility

As the population ages, more patients may enter long-term care facilities. Some are admitted to these facilities for recovery and therapy after an injury or illness. Others are no longer able to care for themselves in their own homes without assistance and will live their remaining months or years in such a facility. Dental hygienists have opportunities to provide care and education in such locations. As patients age or their health deteriorates, it is advantageous for the dental hygienist to provide dental hygiene care in the long-term care facility, rather than stress them with the logistics of scheduling and transporting to the dental office.

The abilities of the patient in the care facility must be assessed before providing oral health care instruction. If it is determined that the patient is not capable of adequate oral hygiene, the caregiver in charge of the patient may be responsible for the oral hygiene. Oral health care education may be provided to groups of long-term care providers through in-service events. Such settings provide opportunities to improve the oral health of their clients. Through education of the importance of preventing oral diseases, by the dental hygienist care providers, will have a better understanding of the need for improved oral health.

Patients in long-term care facilities need daily oral cleansing, whether they have their own teeth or wear dentures. Daily cleansing reduces oral microbes, refreshes the tissues, and helps prevent the accumulation of **sordes,** the crusted accumulation of debris, tissue cells, and microbes that accumulates on the lips, teeth, and oral tissues of helpless or unconscious patients. A damp, soft-bristled toothbrush or power brush is effective for use on these individuals. It may be best to avoid toothpaste if the resulting foam is difficult to manage. Nonfoaming dentifrices that are free of sodium lauryl sulfate, sudsing agent, are available. Dipping the brush in a small amount of fluoride mouthrinse will allow delivery of this caries-preventing agent onto the teeth. During the daily cleansing procedure, care providers can also regularly observe the oral tissues.

The Physically Challenged Patient

Visual Impairment

Dental hygienists rely heavily on visual aids when providing chairside oral health education. Persons with limited visual ability and those with total blindness rely on other senses for image formation and information. Sound and touch can be effective tools in the provision of oral health education of the visually impaired patient. A practical way to approach toothbrush instruction, for example, would be to ask the patient to demonstrate their current brushing technique. With permission, the clinician can position his or her hand over the patient's and guide the toothbrush into the correct position. The individual will *feel* the adaptation of the bristles to the gingival margin. He or she will also *feel* the amount of pressure applied by the clinician to the brush handle and oral tissues. The patient will *feel* and *hear* the bristles as they are activated in small circles or vibratory strokes against the teeth and gingiva.

The same techniques can be applied to instruction on the use of dental floss, with the emphasis placed on how the floss *feels* and *sounds*. Clean tooth surfaces oftentimes squeak, providing the blind patient with immediate information about the effectiveness of their plaque removal efforts. After the dental hygiene care process is complete, ask the visually impaired patient to run their tongue over the tooth surfaces to experience how the surfaces *feel* when plaque-free. They can then try to duplicate that sensation when removing plaque at home as they brush and floss.

Hearing Loss

Hearing loss occurs in varying types and degrees. Some patients lose the ability to hear certain tones. Others note that the voices of some people sound muffled. Some persons have a total loss of hearing ability. This is an obvious impediment to communication in a society that is largely engaged in oral/auditory speech exchanges. Modifications are necessary in order to provide oral hygiene instruction to the dental patient with a hearing impairment.

It may not always be apparent to the dental hygienist that the patient has a hearing loss. Some clues indicating that there is hearing impairment may be lack of response to a question or a response that is not related to the question, frequently asking the speaker to repeat what was said, intently looking at the speaker's face (lips), or a monotone quality of the individual's voice.

Some hearing aids are nearly invisible, and unless the individual tells the clinician, it may go undiscovered. It is important to be aware of the hearing aid for two reasons. First, hearing aids enhance volume and some tones, but wearers of hearing aids generally agree that there is still some hearing loss. The clinician will need to speak clearly and succinctly to aid comprehension. Second, a patient wearing a hearing aid should be instructed to turn it off for power scaling.

Communicating with a person who has a hearing impairment is largely visual. American Sign Language (ASL) is the most-used system of communication for the hearing impaired in the United States (Darby & Walsh, 2003). Clinicians well trained in this system can enrich any dental practice by providing an accurate means of communicating with hearing-impaired patients. However, clinicians that are not well trained in ASL are cautioned when attempting to "sign." Slight gestures and hand position alterations may give unintentional messages, similar to vocal inflections, affecting the intended meaning of verbalized words. Rather than attempt a crash course in ASL, the dental hygienist may want to develop a set of signs that can be readily understood by the clinician and the patient to fit the needs of the particular dental hygiene appointment. Keeping a notepad and pen nearby is helpful as well.

Oral hygiene instructions for the hearing impaired patient can maximize the use of visual information: color flip charts help with identifying the patient's oral condition, radiographs can be used to show areas of alveolar bone loss or interproximal carious lesions, and a disclosing solution will show areas of plaque remaining after brushing and flossing. The patient can use a mirror to watch as correct toothbrushing and flossing techniques are demonstrated. The clinician will want to have his or her mouth visible during communications rather than have it covered by a mask. Persons with hearing loss may be reliant on the visual clues provided by lip movements during speech. The mask that is normally worn by the clinician during dental hygiene care should be off and the clinician should face the listener anytime communication is attempted. Providing the patient with written instructions for personalized oral hygiene can enhance the dental visit and benefits of oral hygiene education.

Muscular, Skeletal, and Nervous System Disorders

Persons with limitations in muscular, skeletal, and/or nervous system function require modification for most of their daily activities. A person without the use of lower extremities may be able to operate an automobile when appropriate modifications to the vehicle have been made. A person without the ability to use his or her hands or arms may still be able to operate a wheelchair that has been modified to allow operation using puffs of air through a mouthpiece. Similarly, the patient with muscular, skeletal, or nervous system disorders may require modifications in oral hygiene instruction and methodologies.

As with all dental health education for the patient, there is no "one size fits all" recommendation for the individual with a physical limitation. It is critical that the patients abilities for self-care be assessed prior to recommending modifications. Whenever possible, the dental hygienist should encourage the patient to take care of his or her own oral hygiene needs; however, some specific tasks may need to be performed by caregivers. Other tasks may be performed by the patient with some modifications that will facilitate self-care.

People with rheumatoid or osteoarthritis involving the finger, hand, wrist, elbow, and/or shoulder joints are likely to have difficulty grasping the handle of a typical toothbrush. The handle can be easily enlarged to allow for a more secure and comfortable grasp. Chapter 8 discusses specific modification ideas. Power brushes are helpful for individuals with a limited range of motion in the hand, wrist, and shoulder areas, but may be too heavy for some (Figure 7.1). The effective use of dental floss is difficult for many. The dental hygienist can consider floss holders or other interproximal aids for the patient with limited manual dexterity (Figure 7.2).

Caregivers that provide assistance in the oral cleansing of those they treat can consider using power toothbrushes for more effectiveness. The rotary and/or vibratory action of the brush head, combined with the larger handle diameter, can prove to be more effective in plaque removal than manual brushing. The floss holder mentioned previously is also another idea for caregivers. Specific instructions can be provided on the use of floss holders in order to avoid lacerations of the patient's gingiva. The floss is held straight and tight between the prongs of the holder. Upon insertion through the contact, the floss must be directed in a mesial or distal direction with an exaggerated "wrap" around the tooth surface, and then the cleansing up-and-down stroke is activated. Failure to adapt to the tooth surface may allow the floss section to traumatize papillary tissue.

Physical Access to Care

As described earlier in the chapter, access to dental care is a mandated right. The physical design of the dental office and understanding the needs of persons with physical limitations will help to make dental care mutually rewarding.

The **Americans with Disabilities Act (ADA)** provides assurance that all individuals will have physical access to services, including dental care. Architectural design guidelines are available through the United States Department of Justice website (www.usdoj.gov/disabilities), which provides specific dimensional requirements for accessibility by persons in wheelchairs. Newer and remodeled facilities are required to be in compliance with the ADA guidelines, but some older dental offices may not be readily accessible. For example, doorways into dental office buildings and individual operatories must be a minimum of 32 inches to accommodate a person in a wheelchair or with a walking frame device (walker). Allowance of 60 inches will enable patients in a wheelchair to execute a 180° turn if needed. Office restrooms and drinking fountains are also evaluated for ease of access by patients with physical disabilities. Provision of such access in the dental office may encourage regular preventive dental care.

The Mentally Challenged Patient

Brain Injury

The human brain is an amazing organ. Science has not yet and may not ever identify the possible functions, abilities, or capacity of the brain. Still, it is a vulnerable organ. Diseases, oxygen deprivation, or chemical or physical injury all have the potential of causing

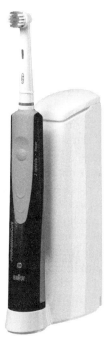

FIGURE 7.1 Oral B-Braun powerbrush.

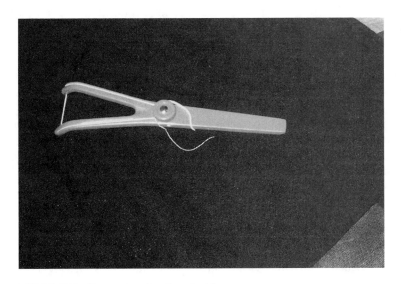

FIGURE 7.2 Example of a floss holder.

irreversible damage. The damage manifests as impairments in sensory, cognitive, and/or motor skills. Dental patients with impairments due to brain injury may also require oral hygiene instruction modifications.

As with the patient with physical challenges, the abilities of patients with mental challenges for self-care must be assessed. It is possible that the patient will be able to adequately remove plaque and debris on a regular basis with some guidance and encouragement. Modifying the toothbrush handle so that it is easier to hold may make the patient's efforts more effective. If it has been determined that the patient with brain injury is not able to adequately remove plaque and debris, oral hygiene instruction can be provided to the caregiver.

The caregiver of the person with a brain injury can be educated to understand that the patient's oral health may also be his or her responsibility as well as the other more obvious duties. Caregivers are often charged with assisting their patients in every aspect of life: feeding, bathing, dressing, transporting, and so on. The dental hygienist's request for them to participate more fully in the patient's oral hygiene may be perceived as an additional burden. Participation and responsibility will be more likely when the caregiver is able to understand the importance of oral health to total well-being.

Mental Retardation

Mental retardation affects people in different ways. A person with mental retardation functions well below average intellectually, with an IQ below 70, and results in challenges for managing life skills (social, communicative, self-care, academic, career, etc.). Levels of mental retardation are based on IQ and function levels: mild, moderate, severe, and profound (Darby & Walsh 2003). (See Table 7.2.) Oral hygiene instructions will be based on the patients level of function.

A person with mild retardation is generally high-functioning, with an IQ between 50 and 70. This person generally lives independently or is lightly supervised, works, and takes care of his or her own personal hygiene needs. Oral hygiene instruction can be based more on the activities involved (brushing and flossing techniques), rather than on the conceptual reasons. The clinician's praise and positive feedback will encourage patient compliance.

A person with moderate retardation has an IQ between 35 and 50. This individual is capable of learning self-care with supervision and reminding. He or she is not able to live or work independently. The person in charge of this patient's care will need to supervise and reinforce oral hygiene efforts. Dental hygienists will want to be alert for signs of frequent fermentable carbohydrate exposure, such as heavy plaque accumulations, gingivitis, and/or multiple carious lesions. Persons with moderate retardation often respond well to positive reinforcement for behavior modification and candy is a favorite "tool" in this technique.

A person with severe retardation has an IQ between 20 and 40. This individual is capable of being trained in some self-care and will require direct oversight. The person with severe retardation usually lives in a group setting, with family or caregivers. Oral hygiene

TABLE 7.2   Levels of Mental Retardation

Level	IQ	Abilities	Dental Hygiene Education
Mild	50–70 (approx.)	Can learn simple skills and self-care.	Teach techniques and activities, not theory
Moderate	35–55 (approx.)	Learns to care for self with supervision and reminding. Responds to positive reinforcement.	Teach individual and caregiver
Severe	20–40 (approx.)	Some self-care with "training" as habit.	Teach individual and caregiver
Profound	Below 20	Dependent on others for self-care. Food preferences increase oral disease risks.	Teach caregiver

instruction takes place with the patient and caregiver. The "training" aspect is habit-based, so it is helpful if the same place, time, technique, and tools are used. Switching toothbrush colors, for example, can be done deliberately and with the patient's involvement, or the change may cause disruption in their habit.

A person with profound retardation has an IQ below 20. This individual is dependant on others for self-care. Oral hygiene instruction is provided to the caregiver, who may encourage limited brushing efforts by the patient. The caregiver must understand that the responsibility for effective plaque removal may be hers/his. Research indicates that individuals with severe to profound retardation have lower amounts of plaque and improved oral health when caregivers are educated in oral hygiene techniques for their patients (Altabet et al., 2003). Soft, sweet, easy-to-chew foods are often preferred by these individuals, placing them at increased risk for caries and gingival/periodontal infections.

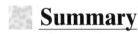 Summary

The patient with special needs may have multiple issues that make getting through an average day challenging. A dental office visit could make that challenging day an exhausting ordeal for the patient with special needs. The dental hygienist has the opportunity and responsibility to understand these special needs and then provide treatment and dental health education modifications. With this understanding, the dental hygienist is able to provide appropriate care in the most pleasant setting possible, the experience can be positive for both the patient and the clinician. A positive dental hygiene care session will encourage regular preventive dental care, reducing the risks of oral disease.

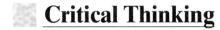 Critical Thinking

1. Describe the consequences of an patient being denied access to dental care.
2. Identify the possible treatment modifications and patient education necessary for the patient with ischemic heart disease.
3. Identify the factors that increase the risk of oral disease in the patient with diabetes.
4. Using Table 7.2, develop an oral hygiene plan for the patient with moderate retardation.
5. Provide the prophylactic antibiotic premedication recommendations for the nonallergic patient.

Activities

1. Using a wheelchair, navigate, using upper body movements only, from your vehicle or clinic entrance to a dental operatory. Notice if the clinic doorways, hallways, and furnishings accommodate movements necessary for negotiating turns required for travel.
2. With a partner, take turns communicating oral health instruction to a patient with visual impairment, and then to a patient with a hearing impairment. Use a scarf to temporarily blindfold or coat safety glasses with petroleum jelly; use a portable music player with ear jacks to interfere with hearing perception.
3. Design oral hygiene instruction methodologies appropriate for the patient with rheumatoid arthritis involving the hands and wrists.
4. Schedule a visit to a group care facility for individuals with mental retardation. Volunteer to develop an oral health care plan for patients living in the facility that includes dental health education for caregivers.

References

Altabet, S., K. Rogers, E. Ines, I. M. Boatman, and J. Moncier. Comprehensive Approach toward Improving Oral Hygiene at a State Residential Facility for People with Mental Retardation. *Mental Retardation*, 41(6) (2003), 440–445.

Centers for Disease Control. *Reported Tuberculosis Cases in the United States, 2002*. Atlanta, GA: Author, 2003.

Darby, M. L., and M. M. Walsh. *Dental Hygiene Theory and Practice*, 2nd ed. Philadelphia: W. B. Saunders, 2003.

Palmer, C. A. *Diet and Nutrition in Oral Health*. Upper Saddle River, NJ: Prentice Hall, 2003.

Requa-Clark, Barbara, *Applied Pharmacology for the Dental Hygienist*, 4th ed. St. Louis: Mosby, 2000.

U.S. Department of Justice. *Americans with Disabilities Act, ADA Title III Technical Assistance Manual.* Washington, DC, 1993.

Wilkins, E. M. *Clinical Practice of the Dental Hygienist,* 9th ed. Baltimore: Lippincott, Williams & Wilkins, 2005.

World Health Organization. *WHO Tuberculosis Fact Sheet Number 104.* Geneva, Switzerland, 2002.

8

Providing Chairside Dental Health Education

Objectives

Upon completion of this chapter, you will be able to

1. Identify individual patient risk factors for development of dental disease.
2. Customize individual patients' oral health education needs based on existing condition.
3. Use effective verbal and nonverbal chairside communication techniques for patient education.
4. Develop an effective chairside dental health education lesson.
5. Develop an effective smoking cessation chairside dental health lesson.

Introduction

Effectively educating the dental hygiene patient may be one of the most overlooked or undervalued areas of dental health care. As previously discussed, the successful outcome (reduction of edema, inflammation, bleeding, pocket depths, etc.) of perfectly executed dental hygiene instrumentation such as periodontal scaling and root planing will be less predictable without regular, effective plaque removal by the patient. Patients' oral health education is based on individual needs, which include existing dental disease, risk for dental disease, abilities and limitations, and willingness to perform oral hygiene tasks.

Achieving excellence in his or her career as a dental hygienist must include ongoing development of instrumentation skill levels, staying abreast of current dental hygiene care modalities, and including patient education in every dental hygiene care session. Dental hygiene care is not complete without effective patient education.

Individualized Dental Health Education

There is no "one size fits all" dental health education speech designed for each patient. The problems presented with such a presentation are many, and include conveying too much information, not enough information, and/or boring the patient to the point of inattention. A patient with periodontal pocket depths generally in excess of 4 mm that bleed on gentle probing has different oral hygiene needs than the patient with rampant caries. Similarly, the continuing care patient with a minuscule amount of plaque without signs of gingival inflammation needs only praise, encouragement, and minor modifications. Information gathered from a variety of sources will help the dental hygienist develop an appropriate patient care plan that includes education for each particular individual.

Dental Disease Risk Assessments

Identification of the patient at risk for developing particular dental diseases is necessary for individualized dental health education. It is critical that the dental hygienist recognize factors that increase a patient's risk of developing periodontal disease or caries, in order to prevent the disease or to arrest disease progression. Recognition of risk includes assessing whether or not that risk is modifiable, and if so, identifying strategies for change. (See Box 8–1.)

Caries Risk

PREVIOUS CARIES HISTORY

The intraoral exam will provide information of current or past caries experience. The patient that has dental caries experience (current carious lesions, restorations or teeth lost due to caries) is considered to be at an increased risk for additional carious lesions (Wilkins, 2005). Areas of demineralization may also indicate an increased caries risk.

The dental hygienist can develop strategies to assist the patient at increased risk of caries. Strategies may include increasing topical fluoride exposure, improving plaque removal, and identifying possible nutritional influences.

OCCLUSAL MORPHOLOGY

Individuals with deep occlusal pits and/or fissures are more likely to develop occlusal carious lesions than those individuals with more shallow occlusal morphology (Wilkins, 2005). These pits and fissures are often visible during the examination, appearing as deeper "trenches" traversing the occlusal surfaces. They may be stained as well. The stains are indicative of the ability of caries-causing bacteria to migrate into pits and fissures. The openings to these pits and fissures are narrower than the bristles of a toothbrush, thus the bacteria remain trapped in the grooves, with the potential of contributing to a carious lesion.

The primary strategy for reducing the risk of caries in the patient with deep occlusal pits and/or fissures is to use sealants, blocking bacterial access (Daniel & Harfst, 2004).

ORAL MEDICATIONS

Frequent exposure to oral medications containing fermentable carbohydrates, such as cough suppressants or lozenges, will increase the patient's risk of caries. Inhaled medications for wheezing and dyspnea with asthma may leave an unpleasant taste in the mouth and patients, particularly children, often relieve the bad taste with candy or beverages high in fermentable carbohydrates.

Strategies to reduce the caries risk resulting from oral medications may include rinsing with water immediately after dosage, improving plaque removal, and multiple topical fluoride exposures by dentifrices, mouthrinses, and topical gel or foam.

MEDICAL CONDITIONS

Diabetes elevates not only the blood glucose, but also the salivary glucose levels. This, combined with xerostomia often found in patients with poorly controlled diabetes, contributes to a higher risk for caries than in the patient whose diabetes is well controlled (Darby & Walsh, 2003). Other medical conditions that cause xerostomia, such as Sjögren's syndrome, salivary gland dysfunction, or cancer therapies, also place the dental patient at risk for caries.

The patient with elevated blood/salivary glucose levels will be encouraged to comply with diet and medication recommendations. Patients not able to control their glucose levels may be referred to their physician. Strategies for the patient with xerostomia resulting from medical conditions or treatments will be discussed later.

FLUORIDE EXPOSURE

Patients choosing to use a nonfluoride dentifrice are at increased risk for caries. Patients that live in communities without a fluoridated water supply do not have the benefit of caries risk reduction via **topical uptake.** Fluoridated water allows frequent **remineralization** opportunities, as do dentifrices and mouthrinses containing fluoride that have been approved by the American Dental Association Council on Dental Therapeutics. This council evaluates the safety and efficacy of dental products before approving them as recommended therapeutic agents. Nonapproved dentifrices and fluoride rinses may contain fluoride formulations that are rendered inactive by the other toothpaste ingredients, thus rendering them ineffective in caries protection.

ORAL HYGIENE

Most dental patients have heard that plaque "causes cavities and gum disease." But most patients are unaware of the effect of plaque on *their* mouths. During the intraoral examination, the dental hygienist will make a determination of the patient's oral hygiene efficacy by the recognition of existing plaque and/or debris and associated inflamed gingival tissue or demineralized enamel. The frequency of brushing and flossing will also affect the amount of plaque and disease. Patients that do not effectively remove dental plaque every 24 hours are at higher risk for caries.

DIETARY HABITS

Frequent exposure to cariogenic foods and/or beverages contributes to a higher risk for caries. (See Chapter 3.) Patients are often unaware of the consequences of seemingly harmless breath mints consumed throughout the day, or sipping on sweetened coffee or tea all morning. While these practices may not contribute much to the patient's daily caloric intake, the constant "feeding" of the plaque bacteria will contribute to thicker, more virulent plaque.

ACCESS TO DENTAL CARE

Consumers may have difficulty obtaining the dental care they need due to transportation challenges, financial limitations, or lack of dental insurance. Chapter 1 discusses these obstacles; Chapter 7 describes more of the barriers for patients with special needs. Limited access to dental care impedes regular, preventative dental services. Dental diseases such as caries and periodontal disease are less likely to be treated in a proactive manner. Patients with limited access are more prone to emergency services only.

Periodontal Disease Risk

TABACCO USE

The link between tobacco use and periodontal disease has been clearly established. Patients that smoke are approximately three times more likely to have compromised periodontal health with the accompanying loss of attachment and increased periodontal pocket depths (Johnson & Hill, 2004). Patients using chewing (spit) tobacco are at risk for gingival recession. Dental hygienists are better equipped to provide education when aware of whether or not their patient is currently using tobacco products and if so, the quantity and frequency of use.

DIETARY FACTORS

Similar to caries risk, periodontal disease is more likely to occur and be difficult to control in the patient that experiences frequent fermentable carbohydrate exposure. In addition, inadequate intakes of key nutrients such as protein and zinc will contribute to an increase in the severity of the periodontal condition. Rapidly destructive gingival diseases such as **acute necrotizing ulcerative periodontal (diseases) ANUP** are particularly exacerbated by a deficiency in vitamin C (AAP, 2004).

SYSTEMIC FACTORS

Patients with medical conditions such as diabetes, rheumatoid arthritis, osteoporosis, and pregnancy are at higher risk for developing periodontal disease (AAP). Early recognition and intervention by the dental hygienist is necessary for successful treatment of the periodontal condition. In addition, active periodontal disease contributes to blood glucose regulation difficulties for the diabetic patient (Taylor, 2001). Also, the link between periodontal disease and the development of cardiovascular diseases and coronary heart disease. Recent studies have shown some encouraging news for those patients with osteoporosis and osteopenia. Some patients being treated with estrogen replacement therapy and nutritional supplements, usually calcium and vitamin D, showed reductions in their rates of alveolar bone loss (Krall, 2001).

MEDICATIONS

The use of medications such as Dilantin, steroids, cancer therapies, calcium channel blockers, and contraceptives increases the risk and severity of periodontal disease (ADA, 1995–2004).

FAMILY HISTORY

Patients who have had one or both parents experience periodontal disease are at increased risk for periodontal disease (ADA, 1995–2004). This familial link is genetic, but may also include cultural and/or social factors that are learned.

PREVIOUS PERIODONTAL TREATMENT

Patients that have had periodontal disease requiring treatment are at risk for future periodontal disease. This is due, in part, to the loss of gingival attachment and alveolar bone. Successful periodontal treatments will arrest the progression, but will not restore the attachment or bone without bone and/or tissue grafts. A second aspect of this risk is that the factors contributing to periodontal disease, such as a lack of host resistance to the disease (nonmodifiable) or tobacco use (modifiable), may still be present.

BLEEDING ON PROBING

This is the hallmark sign of gingival/periodontal disease as observed by the dental hygienist. Bleeding on probing is an indication of active disease. The dental patient with this clinical sign is at risk for loss of attachment and alveolar bone.

ORAL HYGIENE

Failure to effectively and regularly remove bacterial plaque from the dental surfaces, embrasure and sulcular spaces, and proximal surfaces will increase the patient's risk of gingi-

Box 8–1 Sampling of oral disease risk factors and strategies.

Modifiable	Non-modifiable	Strategy
	Previous caries/perio disease	Patient education
Occlusal morphology		Pit and fissure sealants
Xerostomia		Increase fluoride exposure
	Medical conditions	Patient education
Non-fluoridated water source		Increase fluoride exposure
Inadequate oral hygiene		Patient education
Frequent sugar consumption		Patient education
Tobacco use		Patient education
	Family history of oral disease	Patient education

val/periodontal disease. The patient presenting with observable areas of plaque accumulation or admitting to brushing and flossing irregularly may be presumed to be at high risk for a periodontal disease.

Risk Assessments

In 2004 Dr. Randy Rolf introduced a risk calculating software program (PreViser) designed for dental practices that would allow the dental hygienist to become more accurate in their risk assessing skills, yet more importantly, provide the patient with a risk result based on their past and current habits. These risk assessments were developed for caries as well as periodontal disease. The caries risk assessment process was broken down even further to address specific age groups. PreViser also spent 10 years in clinical trials before releasing their software to dental professionals. The results of these clinical trials can be found in the *Journal of Clinical Periodontology* and the *Journal of the American Dental Association.* A sample of the PreViser caries risk assessment form is seen in Figure 8.1. The periodontal disease risk assessment form is seen in Figure 8.2. For more information on this software, visit the website at http://www.previser.com.

Evaluating the Patient's Oral Hygiene

Accumulations of plaque are easily recognizable by the experienced dental hygienist, but the average patient may be unaware. The dull appearance of their enamel or rough feel of their teeth to their tongue may seem normal. An effective tool for demonstrating the patient's plaque removal effectiveness is a **plaque index.** A plaque index is a tool that can be very useful for patient education. A patient's perception of their plaque removal efforts is often quite different than what is revealed by measuring the percentage of tooth surfaces containing plaque. A method for the determining the patient's plaque percentage has been developed by O'Leary, Drake, and Naylor (1972). This can be modifiable in order to suit the needs of the patient, clinic, or office. Every tooth surface is evaluated. Whether to evaluate four or six surfaces per tooth is determined in advance. A diagram showing individual teeth divided into segments of four or six will aid in the calculation of the patient's plaque score. (See Figure 8.3.) A disclosing solution is applied to the patient's teeth. The dental hygienist will mark the diagram on each tooth surface showing disclosed plaque, and then total them. The number of teeth being observed is multiplied by the number of surfaces on each tooth being observed, four or six. The total number of tooth surfaces with plaque is divided by the number of surfaces being observed. That number is multiplied by 100 to give a percentage score:

$$\frac{\text{Total surfaces with plaque}}{\text{4 or 6} \times \text{number of teeth in mouth}} \times 100 = \text{plaque percentage}$$

A plaque score of 0% is ideal, but unlikely. A score of 10% or below is usually considered desirable for successful periodontal treatment success. Patients are often surprised when

Caries Risk Analysis Input Form - Patient Age 34 and Older

Prepared by

Prepared for

Name: _____

Date of Birth: _____

Internal Patient ID: _____

Previser Patient ID: _____

Exam Date: _____

Last Assessment Date: _____

Patient History and Clinical Data

Permanent premolars and molars
a) Sound or sealed
b) Carious or early decalcification
c) 1–2 interproximal restorations
d) >2 interproximal restorations

Root surfaces
a) Not visible
b) Visible and sound
c) Carious
d) Restored

Months Patient has been Caries free
a) 36 or more
b) 24–35
c) 12–23
d) Less than 12

☐ Erosion, abrasion, or abfraction on Root Surface

☐ A tooth has been fractured

☐ A tooth that is present has root canal fillings and is not restored with a crown

Oral Hygiene
Excellent: improvement not possible
Acceptable: slight improvement possible
Unacceptable: substantial improvement needed

☐ Fluoride products are used (Fluoridated water, toothpaste, rinses or gels)

☐ Has fixed orthodontic appliance

☐ Experiences dry mouth

☐ Bruxes, grinds, or clenches.
- OR -
Symptoms of habits like occlusal or incisal wear, tooth facets, or cervical wear exist

☐ Has a pierced tongue or oral habits like eating ice, playing a musical instrument with a mouthpiece, or opening a bottle that places excessive stress on the teeth

☐ Has had a major change in health (heart attack, stroke, etc.) during the past 12 months

a) 5 or More
b) 4 or Less

Times per day snacks or beverages containing sugar are consumed between meals

Treatments Performed since last Risk Assessment

Preventive Treatment

Prophylaxis/Maintenance	☐ # procedures	Nutritional counseling/referral	☐ # times
Sealants	☐ # teeth	Tobacco counseling/referral	☐ # times
Topical fluoride	☐ # procedures	Medical condition referral	☐ # times
Oral hygiene instruction	☐ # procedures	Oral habit instruction	☐ # times
		Bite guard	☐ # procedures

Related to Teeth

Restorations	☐ # teeth
Endodontics	☐ # teeth

Related to Periodontium

Systemic chemotherapy	☐ # times
Local delivery - chemotherapy	☐ # sites
Scaling and root planing	☐ # quadrants
Surgery-pockets, vertical bone, furcas	☐ # quadrants
Surgery-pockets, vertical bone, furcas	☐ # procedures
Surgery-other	☐ # quadrants
Surgery-other	☐ # procedures

Related to Tooth Replacement

Extractions	☐ # teeth
Single tooth replacement - implants	☐ # implants
Fixed prosthesis	☐ # prostheses
Teeth abutments	☐ # teeth
Implant abutments	☐ # implants
Pontics	☐ # pontics
Removable prosthesis	☐ # prostheses
Implant abutments	☐ # implants
Provisional splinting	☐ # teeth+pontics

FIGURE 8.1 Previser Caries Risk Analysis.

Periodontal Risk and Disease Analysis Input Form

Prepared by

Prepared for

Name: _____

Date of Birth: _____

Internal Patient ID: _____

Previser Patient ID: _____

Exam Date: _____

Last Assessment Date: _____

Patient History and Clinical Data

Dental Care Frequency	Smoking History	Diabetic
a) Unknown b) Never/First visit c) 1–2 per year d) >2 per year e) Irregular f) Emergency	a) Unknown b) Never smoked c) Former smoker d) Smokes <10 per day e) Smokes >=10 per day	a) Unknown b) Not diabetic c) Good diabetic control d) Fair diabetic control e) Poor diabetic control

☐ Periodontal Surgery for Pockets Has Been Done

☐ Bleeding on Probing

☐ Furcation Involvements

☐ Defective Subgingival Restorations

☐ Vertical Bone Lesions

☐ Calculus on Radiographs or Below the Gingival Margin

Oral Hygiene

a) Excellent: improvement not possible
b) Acceptable: slight improvement possible
c) Unacceptable: substantial improvement needed

Pocket Depths

Upper Right	Upper Anterior	Upper Left
a) <5 mm b) 5–7 mm c) >7 mm d) No Teeth	a) <5 mm b) 5–7 mm c) >7 mm d) No Teeth	a) <5 mm b) 5–7 mm c) >7 mm d) No Teeth

Lower Right	Lower Anterior	Lower Left
a) <5 mm b) 5–7 mm c) >7 mm d) No Teeth	a) <5 mm b) 5–7 mm c) >7 mm d) No Teeth	a) <5 mm b) 5–7 mm c) >7 mm d) No Teeth

Radiographic Bone Height from CEJ

Upper Right	Upper Anterior	Upper Left
a) <2 mm b) 2–4 mm c) >4 mm d) No Teeth	a) <2 mm b) 2–4 mm c) >4 mm d) No Teeth e) No X-Ray	a) <2 mm b) 2–4 mm c) >4 mm d) No Teeth

Lower Right	Lower Anterior	Lower Left
a) <2 mm b) 2–4 mm c) >4 mm d) No Teeth	a) <2 mm b) 2–4 mm c) >4 mm d) No Teeth e) No X-Ray	a) <2 mm b) 2–4 mm c) >4 mm d) No Teeth

Treatments Performed since last Risk Assessment

Preventive Treatment

Prophylaxis/Maintenance	☐ # procedures	Nutritional counseling/referral	☐ # times
Sealants	☐ # teeth	Tobacco counseling/referral	☐ # times
Topical fluoride	☐ # procedures	Medical condition referral	☐ # times
Oral hygiene instruction	☐ # procedures	Oral habit instruction	☐ # times
		Bite guard	☐ # procedures

Related to Teeth

Restorations ☐ # teeth

Endodontics ☐ # teeth

Related to Periodontium

Systemic chemotherapy ☐ # times

Local delivery - chemotherapy ☐ # sites

Scaling and root planing ☐ # quadrants

Surgery-pockets, vertical bone, furcas ☐ # quadrants

Surgery-pockets, vertical bone, furcas ☐ # procedures

Surgery-other ☐ # quadrants

Surgery-other ☐ # procedures

Related to Tooth Replacement

Extractions ☐ # teeth

Single tooth replacement - implants ☐ # implants

Fixed prosthesis ☐ # prostheses

  Teeth abutments ☐ # teeth

  Implant abutments ☐ # implants

  Pontics ☐ # pontics

Removable prosthesis ☐ # prostheses

  Implant abutments ☐ # implants

Provisional splinting ☐ # teeth+pontics

FIGURE 8.2 Previser Periodontal Risk Analysis.

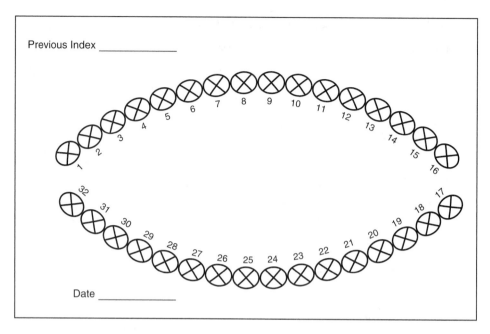

Previous Index _____

Date _____

FIGURE 8.3 Sample of plaque index diagram or form.

their scores are 25% or higher. The disclosed plaque and diagram are also effective for demonstrating areas missed by the toothbrush and/or dental floss.

The dental hygienist should not assume that the patient with a plaque percentage of 40% is not trying to effectively remove plaque. It would be inappropriate to begin the oral hygiene instructions providing toothbrush and floss demonstrations without first evaluating the patient's existing technique. The patient may become defensive or resistant when the "correct way to brush your teeth" is demonstrated. The patient may be aware of the "correct way" but has been rushing through their oral hygiene. Asking the patient to "show me how you normally brush your teeth" may provide insights to modification needs.

The Oral Hygiene Education Plan

Upon clinical assessment of the patient, the dental hygienist will be equipped to formulate a customized, individualized oral hygiene education plan for each patient. The information provided guides and directs the development of this plan. Factors may include but are not limited to:

- Patient's oral health status (gingivitis, periodontitis, caries, health)
- Patient's risk assessments (gingivitis, periodontitis, caries)
- Patient's current oral hygiene status

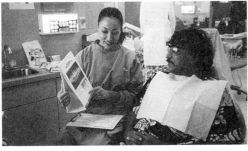
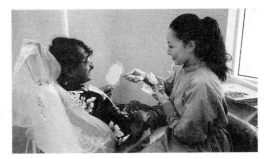

A   **B**

FIGURE 8.4   Dental hygienist providing chairside oral hygiene instruction.

- Patient's "hot button" or reason for the motivation to change (see Chapters 5 and 6)
- "Dental IQ" or current understanding of oral condition and consequences

Chairside Communication

As described in Chapter 4, communication skills is critical for effective oral health education. The dental hygienist will utilize his or her understanding of verbal and nonverbal communication techniques for enhanced understanding of the patient's needs and abilities. Active listening is a critical aspect of this communication. Restating often leads to clarification and avoids misunderstanding (feedback).

It may be helpful for the dental hygienist to think of the oral hygiene education session as a mutually informative conversation rather than a one-sided lecture session, thus the physical aspects of this *dialogue* is important. The patient should be in an upright position for oral hygiene education. Placing the patient at eye level is often more conducive for comfortable exchange of information. This is even more critical when working with a patient that is fearful or anxious. The clinician's mask, eye protection, and gloves can be eliminated at this point, allowing the patient to see and hear the clinician.

The following items can be accessible during the oral hygiene education session:

- Patient's periodontal chart
- Patient's current bite-wing and full mouth radiographs
- Toothbrush, dental floss, and other oral hygiene aids selected for patient
- Flip-chart or other visual tools showing stages of health and disease
- Disclosing solution and plaque index diagram
- Hand-held mirror for patient

The following is a sample dialogue demonstrating an oral hygiene education session between a dental hygienist (DH) and patient (Mrs. Smith):

DH: Mrs. Smith, as I was describing earlier, I have been evaluating your oral health condition by examining your "gum" tissues and x-rays, and measuring the pocket depths and plaque amounts. What I have found today shows me that you have an early form of periodontal disease and I'd like to help you deal with it right away. Have you ever been told before that you had periodontal disease?

Mrs. Smith: No, but I've been thinking about it. When you asked me earlier about my family history of periodontal disease, I realized that my mother lost her teeth in her early forties. I never knew why because my mother had beautiful teeth and never had any fillings. Does this mean I'll need dentures, too?

DH: I think we can avoid that, Mrs. Smith, because we're catching this condition early. See these x-rays? If you look right here you can see the level of the bone that supports your teeth. And right here is where it started before being affected by periodontal disease. If this condition continues without treatment, the bone will keep migrating toward the end of the "root," until the periodontal condition is so severe that some teeth may be lost. When I measured your pockets with my periodontal probe, I found depths between 4 and 5 millimeters. Most of those areas bled when I probed, showing me that the disease is active.

Mrs. Smith: What do we need to do to stop it?

DH: I'm glad you said "we" because that's how this will work, as a partnership. I'll thoroughly clean the surfaces of the teeth and roots and then you'll need to keep the plaque off of those surfaces regularly. We both have to do a good job, or the disease may not be stopped. If you look at this picture, it shows a cross-section of a tooth in the supporting bone. This tooth has "tartar" on its root surfaces. We call that tartar calculus. The calculus holds onto bacterial plaque that is difficult to reach. The plaque's byproducts contribute to the progression of the disease, so when it is trapped on calculus, the condition gets worse. Your teeth have calculus on the roots too, and I'll need to remove that with my instruments. Then . . .

Mrs. Smith: I know. Then I'll need to do my part. If I keep the plaque off will the calculus come back?

DH: Great question, Mrs. Smith. Plaque is continuously reforming on your teeth and when it's not regularly removed it can mineralize and become calculus. But if you start doing your best plaque removal right after I clean your teeth and roots, I expect a good healing response. The "swollen gum" tissue should firm up against the bone, shrinking the pockets. The pockets will be smaller and more "cleanable" by you. With your good oral hygiene and regular maintenance visits here, your periodontal condition can be arrested.

Mrs. Smith: I'd like to get started right away. Please show me what I need to do.

DH: Okay. I used that red disclosing solution to show me how much plaque was on your teeth. I found that 30% of your tooth surfaces had plaque on them.

Mrs. Smith: 30% sounds pretty good doesn't it? That means that 70% of my teeth are clean, right?

DH: It would seem like that wouldn't it? But we know that for a good healing response to occur, we'll need a plaque score of 10% or less. Let's see what we can do to get your score down.

The fictitious patient above is ready for toothbrush and floss instruction. The disclosing solution used for the plaque index is also a good indicator of areas the patient may tend to miss when brushing or flossing. The dental hygienist can observe these tendencies and show them to the patient with the hand mirror. Then the sequence may go as follows:

- Patient is asked to demonstrate their current toothbrushing method
- Clinician observes and makes positive observations
- Clinician demonstrates modifications needed
- Patient demonstrates, applying new modifications
- Clinician observes and remodifies if necessary

The same technique can be used for dental floss instruction as well as any other aids, such as interproximal brushes or picks. It should be noted that in the dialogue the dental hygienist provides positive communication, even when correction is necessary.

Motivation and Learning

In the above illustration, the patient, Mrs. Smith, is already motivated to become an active participant in improving her oral health. She was beginning to have some concerns about losing her teeth as her mother had, and was a receptive learner. She was eager to learn how to do her part in stopping her periodontal disease. But what about the patient that is not very receptive to the information and education? Recall from Chapters 5 and 6 the different ages, stages, and influences on patients. Through active communication and an understanding of these varying phases, the dental hygienist is able to discover a motivating "hot button." The pregnant woman with gingivitis may be motivated to improve her oral health when she understands that the health of her unborn baby may be affected. The adolescent may be interested in improving the appearance of his or her smile.

Oral Hygiene Modifications

Some patients are not able to use a toothbrush or floss effectively. When the patient is asked to demonstrate their technique, it may become apparent that some modifications can be made to improve plaque removal. Chapter 7 discusses several factors that may inhibit plaque removal efforts and modifications to accommodate them.

It may also become necessary to modify recommendations when the patient will not or cannot use a certain item for plaque removal. Some patients simply will not use dental floss regularly, even after repeated oral health education sessions. The dental hygienist should not presume that the patient is doomed to interproximal caries and/or gingival disease. Other interproximal devices may be implemented, such as interproximal brushes or wooden picks.

Tobacco Use Cessation

Tobacco use is a major contributor to compromised oral and systemic health. The dental hygienist plays a key role in the support system for the smoker who wants to quit. Most individuals know that cigarette smoking causes various health challenges, including increased risk of cancer, preterm low birth weight babies, and cardiovascular disease. The dental patient may be unaware of tobacco's contribution to oral disease, including periodontal disease and oral cancer. The dental hygienist may be the health care provider to provide the information necessary which motivates the patient to stop smoking.

Education is the key to motivation, with tobacco use cessation as well as other modifications in self-care. Smokers are bombarded from many angles with reasons to quit: the media, the cost of cigarettes, their family, even government regulations banning smoking in many public areas. A careful approach may therefore be necessary when discussing this topic with the dental patient in order to avoid defensiveness, resentment, or even anger. Such negative responses may imped communication and patient education opportunity.

Researchers with the National Cancer Institute (2004) have concluded that "Based on good evidence, counseling by a health professional improves smoking cessation." The National Cancer Institute, in conjunction with the Agency for Healthcare Research and Quality (AHRQ), developed a model for use by healthcare workers when treating patients who use tobacco. This model, *Five Major Steps to Intervention (The "5A's")* (2000), is readily applicable to chairside dental health education. The five major steps are:

1. **Ask**—find out the tobacco use status for each patient at every visit.
2. **Advise**—firmly urge every tobacco user to quit.
3. **Assess**—determine the willingness of the tobacco user to quit at this time.
4. **Assist**—for the willing patient, use counseling or recommend pharmacotherapy to help him or her quit.
5. **Arrange**—plan a follow-up contact (such as a phone call), preferably within the first week after the prearranged quit date.

The "assist" aspect of this model also has guidelines for counseling. AHRQ has divided these counseling guidelines for helping patients to quit into practical advice:

- **Recognize danger situations**—advise patients that certain events, emotions, or activities will increase the risk of relapse.
- **Develop coping skills**—assist the patient in identifying and practicing skills that will help him or her cope with danger situations.
- **Provide basic information**—the patient should be informed of health risks associated with tobacco use, periodontal tissue effects, and the symptoms and duration of nicotine withdrawal.
- **Encourage the patient in the quit attempt**—the dental hygienist may be the "you can do this!" cheerleader. The patient will be encouraged to know that over half of all of the people that have smoked have now quit.

- **Communicate caring and concern**—the patient may appreciate being asked how he or she feels about quitting. The dental hygienist may show concern and willingness to help, while being open to the patient's expressed fears and difficulties with quitting.
- **Encourage the patient to talk about the quitting process**—the dental hygienist may ask about the reasons the patient wants to quit, their concerns about quitting, or their successes and difficulties while quitting, for example.

Additional information and support tools are available on the websites for the National Cancer Institute (www.nci.nih.gov) and the Agency for Healthcare Research and Quality (www.ahrq.gov.)

The bulk of this information has been concerned with tobacco use in the form of cigarettes, as most patients that use tobacco smoke. The users of chewing (spit) tobacco can also be assisted in their efforts to quit. Orally absorbed tobacco products and nicotine are harmful and highly addictive. These patients will need the same caring support as patient using cigarettes.

Summary

Patient education is one of the most rewarding and challenging aspects of dental hygiene care. To effectively educate the dental patient, many factors must be considered, including the current dental health status, risk factors affecting their dental health, the current level of plaque removal efficacy, limitations that may prevent optimal oral hygiene, and the willingness to participate in improving their oral health status.

Clinical skills alone are not enough for optimal dental health. Active participation by the patient involves more than showing up for their appointments. The dental hygienist is charged with the responsibility of providing education of the patient's dental condition, the necessary treatment for that condition, and the role of the patient in modifying that condition. Patient education draws on the clinician's understanding of positive communication skills and patient motivation, as well as the ability to modify recommendations to fit the individual patient's needs and limitations.

Critical Thinking

1. Describe the modifiable risk factors for periodontal disease. Suggest modifications for those risks.
2. Describe the modifiable risk factors for caries. Suggest modifications for those risks.
3. Explain the use of a plaque index in patient education.
4. Suggest oral hygiene recommendations for the dental patient with rheumatoid arthritis that is unable to grasp a traditional toothbrush or hold dental floss.
5. List the harmful effects of tobacco use, including oral and systemic.

Activities

1. With a student partner, identify each other's risks for caries and periodontal disease, determine their plaque score, and develop a personalized oral hygiene education plan.

2. In small groups, consider the following patient cases. Identify modifiable risks for periodontal disease, suggest modifications, and develop a personalized plan for dental hygiene care and oral hygiene education. Present each group's recommendations and discuss similarities, differences, and rationale for those recommendations:

Case application 1: John is a 45-year-old Hispanic male, height 5'10", weight 220 pounds. His blood pressure is in the prehypertensive range. He was diagnosed with Type 2 diabetes 1 year ago and states that he tries to keep it managed with diet and exercise. He smokes one pack of cigarettes per day. He works in outside sales and eats "on the run." His days are long and he states that he depends on cola beverages for the caffeine boost. His father had "great teeth" but had them removed at age 40 because they were "getting loose." Clinical examination reveals radiographic evidence of vertical bone loss, generalized 4 to 5mm pocket depths, generalized bleeding on probing, localized 2mm recession on buccal surfaces of #13, 14, 19, 28, 29, and 30. Subgingival calculus deposits are moderate with some interproximal "spurs." John's plaque index score is 42% with the predominance of plaque located on interproximal surfaces.

Case application 2: Rose is a 62-year-old Caucasian female, height is 5'3", weight 130 pounds. Her blood pressure is within the normal range. She was diagnosed with osteoporosis 2 years ago and takes Fosamax® once weekly as directed. She takes calcium supplements, 1200 mg per day. She teaches piano lessons to four students each week. She tries not to go outside during peak sun hours to protect her skin. She drinks hot tea in the morning only, sweetened with Splenda®. Living alone, she says she rarely prepares complete meals and prefers to snack on her favorite foods off and on all day. Ms. Davis was adopted at age 2 and did not know her birth parents. Clinical examination reveals radiographic evidence of moderate horizontal bone loss, 3 to 4mm pocket depths with no bleeding on probing, generalized buccal and lingual 2 to 3mm recession. Subgingival calculus is slight, with light supragingival calculus on the lingual proximal surfaces of the lower anterior teeth. Her plaque index score is 18% with the predominance of plaque located on the lingual surfaces.

References

Agency for Healthcare Research and Quality. *Treating Tobacco Use and Dependence, Public Health Services Clinical Practice Guideline: Five Major Steps to Intervention (The 5 A's)/Counseling Patients to Quit.* http://www.ahrq.gov, 2000.

American Academy of Periodontology. *Oral Health Information for the Public: Gum Disease.* http://www.perio.org, 2004.

American Dental Association. *Oral Health Topics: Periodontal Disease.* http://www.ada .org, 1995–2004.

Daniel, S. J., and S. A. Harfst. *Dental Hygiene Concepts, Cases, and Competencies.* St. Louis, MO: Mosby, 2004.

Darby, M. L., and M. M. Walsh. *Dental Hygiene Theory and Practice*, 2nd ed. Philadelphia: W. B. Saunders, 2003.

De Nardin, E. The Role of Inflammatory and Immunological Mediators in Periodontitis and Cardiovascular Disease. *Annals of Periodontology, 6*(1) (2001).

Johnson, G. K., and M. Hill. Cigarette Smoking and the Periodontal Patient. *Journal of Periodontology, 75* (2004).

Krall, E. A. The Periodontal-Systemic Connection: Implications for Treatment of Patients with Osteoporosis and Periodontal Disease. *Annals of Periodontology, 6*(1) (2001).

National Cancer Institute. *Prevention and Cessation of Cigarette Smoking: Control of Tobacco Use.* http://www.nci.nih.gov/cancertopics/pdq, 2004.

O'Leary, T. J., R. B. Drake, and J. E. Naylor. The Plaque Control Record. *Journal of Periodontology, 43* (1972), 38.

Taylor, G. W. Bidirectional Interrelationships between Diabetes and Periodontal Diseases: An Epidemiologic Perspective. *Annals of Periodontology, 6*(1) (2001).

Wilkins, E. M. *Clinical Practice of the Dental Hygienist*, 9th ed. Baltimore: Lippincott, Williams & Wilkins, 2005.

9

Education for Community Populations

Objectives

Upon reading the material in this chapter, you will be able to

1. Discuss standard of care for dental hygiene procedures.
2. Identify professional responsibilities to patients.
3. Discuss responsibility to the dental hygiene profession.
4. List basic human needs for oral health.
5. Prepare dental health lessons for a specific population group.

Introduction

As dental hygiene students, professionalism, responsibility, and duty to patient care rank high in the educational process. Upon licensure, these responsibilities expand to include employers, coworkers, communities, colleagues, and the professional association. Many practitioners often overlook these aspects of the dental hygiene career; however, it is wise to keep them in the forefront while developing into a professional health care provider. There are certain expectations by all who interact with the dental hygienist, and vice versa. Oral health is a need for all humans, yet everyone is at a different level of need. As a licensed health care provider, it will be beneficial to explore and participate in all aspects of the dental hygiene profession.

Basic Human Needs

Initial thoughts for basic human needs might include food, water, clothing, and shelter. And although these are needs for all persons, there are basic needs regarding oral health that may not come to mind as quickly or as easily. Oftentimes, dental health care workers share stories that include how they have become more observant of teeth once they have entered the field. Upon gaining more knowledge and experience as a dental assistant, front office worker, and especially a dental hygiene student, the size, shape, position, color, and condition of teeth in everyone we meet and talk with become a focal point. Over decades of improved technology, oral health clinicians still find high decay rates, lack of orthodontic attention, lack of preventive measures by consumers for plaque and calculus control, and amazingly enough, lack of patient compliance for home care recommended by the dental hygienist. As already pointed out, economic trends and levels have influenced the consumer's ability to afford quality dental care for far too many families in the United States, yet technology has not decreased caries rates in young children, and periodontal diseases overall. Thus, as dental professionals, it is a duty to recognize basic needs for oral health so that the general public benefits from the education and the services available to them in their community.

What is meant by basic human needs when it comes to oral health? Michele Darby and Margaret Walsh have been recognized for developing a conceptual model that considers several factors as related to dental health, such as a human need, a cause, or etiology as related to the patient's current oral condition.

These basic needs include the following:

- Safety—freedom from harm or danger
- Freedom from pain/stress—exemption from physical and emotional discomforts
- Wholesome body image—positive mental representation of one's own body
- Skin and mucous membrane integrity of the head and neck
- Nutrition—the need for a balanced diet
- A biologically sound dentition—need for intact teeth and restorations that provide function
- Conceptualization and problem solving—to grasp ideas and make sound judgments
- Appreciation and respect—need for acknowledgment and achievements
- Self-determination and responsibility—need to exercise firmness of purpose about one's self and behavior
- Territoriality—to possess a prescribed area of space or knowledge
- Value system—freedom to develop one's own sense of importance

(*Source:* Kimbrough & Lautar, 2003)

How do these basic needs apply to dental hygiene education? Let's look at one of the human needs listed, "a biologically sound dentition," and create a case scenario.

Case Scenario 1:

Mr. B is having his dental hygiene treatment with you for the first time, and he has not been in the office for an exam for 6 years. After talking with him for a few minutes, you take a quick look into his mouth and see two areas where the tooth crowns have fractured and are missing. Upon new radiographs taken that day, you also notice areas with carious lesions, yet to be evaluated by the dentist. In reviewing his dental history with the practice, you notice that he was very regular with his preventive visits and annual examinations.

   1. What may have occurred to change his dental care pattern?
   2. How does he value his dentition in the long term?
   3. Have there been changes in diet? Economy? Dental insurance coverage?
   4. What does he want with regard to his oral health?

The case presented also includes some questions that may be appropriate to ask the patient. In attempting to determine why the oral condition exists in its current state, the practitioner will want to be sure he or she understands any possible change in Mr. B's lifestyle that may have been an influence.

By recognizing some of these basic human needs, and understanding that there are many factors that contribute to the current conditions of every patient, the dental hygienist can play a major role in determining how to design the appropriate approach and treatment plan. When students and practitioners are aware of what is valued by the patient and how they view themselves and their oral health, the dental hygiene treatment plan can incorporate appropriate oral hygiene aids, etiology discussion, home care therapy, and continuing care intervals. The clinician can also assist in identifying what type of restorations or esthetic desires the patient may be interested in and relay that information to the dentist. The dental hygienist can also ensure that the appropriate specialist is contacted when needed. Most importantly, being able to identify oral health needs and the values of each patient helps to establish rapport and professionalism. There is no "canned" version of oral health care and recommendations. Each patient is unique in their needs, perceptions, values, and conditions. This uniqueness is why dental hygienists find their career both rewarding and exciting: nothing is ever the same.

Duties to the Patient

As licensed practitioners, there are duties to uphold with regard to the laws of the license, as well as the ethical standards of the profession. As patients or clients, the consumer has certain rights that must be acknowledged and respected by the practitioner. There are recognized standards of care for all aspects of healthcare as well. For example, when the dental consumer agrees to a restorative procedure, like a composite filling, the patient expects the dentist to prepare and restore the tooth using standard techniques taught in dental school, and using the appropriate materials. Similarly, dental hygienists have a duty to uphold the **standard of care** for dental hygiene procedures, radiographs, and oral health education to the same degree as any other dental health care provider. In other words, it is care that any reasonably prudent person would exercise under the same or similar circumstances. The profession and professionals themselves develop these standards (Darby & Walsh, 1995). Standards can become engrained as part of the profession when practiced and upheld by all members of the profession. They are not laws, and are not viewed as laws by the courts should a lawsuit occur between a consumer and the health care provider. When lawsuits do occur, it is likely, and most commonly due to negligence on the part of the practitioner, due to a breach in the standard of care. Thus, when the lawsuit goes before a judge or a jury, experts or practitioners in the same field may be called upon to provide adequate information to substantiate the case.

Reasonable standard of care for dental hygiene may include but may not be limited to taking vitals, updating the medical information, informing the patient of their condition, and keeping current dental documents such as radiographs and periodontal charting. When the dental hygienist does not uphold standards, lawsuits can occur. Maintaining high-quality patient care in all working environments will ensure that the consumer receives what is expected from the professional, and avoid potential litigation.

Other duties to the patient include ethical core values. This text is not designed to present ethics in detail, however, basic values are included in Table 9.1.

Ethical principles and values are significant in dental hygiene as well as all health care professions. These principles assist in the foundation for high-quality patient care and education. Consumers expect that their health care provider is a member of their respective professional association. From the consumers' perspective, this membership signifies that the practitioner holds high values in all aspects of their field. It means they are staying current with new technology in health care. Dentists and physicians often include in their advertising the fellowships they hold, that they are a member of specific societies or associations related to their field of expertise. This indicates to consumers that they are well networked and respected among colleagues. The dental hygienist has a duty to the patient to be an active member in his or her professional association. Consumers are unaware of the extensive education the dental hygienist can hold. There are many clinicians

TABLE 9.1 Core Values of the ADHA Code of Ethics

Autonomy	To guarantee self-determination of the patient
Confidentiality	To hold in confidence secret information entrusted by the patient
Societal trust	To ensure the trust patients and society have in dental hygienists
Nonmaleficence	To do no harm to the patient
Beneficence	To benefit the patient
Justice	To benefit the patient
Veracity	To tell the truth, not to lie to the patient

Source: Kimbrough & Lautar, 2003

that have obtained master's degrees and doctorate degrees, yet the consumer has no idea. The education and professional membership of the dental hygienist is just as significant as that of dentists and physicians. It will be up to the practitioner to inform their patient as part of building rapport and mutual respect.

Duties to the Profession

Many states require postgraduate continuing education units for licensed professionals. This means that the clinician continues to take educational courses or seminars to stay updated on technology, procedures, and materials. From a professional standpoint this is essential. As practitioners network in their communities, current knowledge on dental hygiene technology will enhance patient care and education. When designing an oral health seminar for school children, teens, adults, caregivers, or fellow professionals, incorporating the latest materials and procedures assist in improving oral health for all. Here again, professional membership plays a significant role in keeping all licensed practitioners updated on their chosen career.

Many dental practices often employ more than one dental hygienist. When working with a colleague, it provides a greater opportunity to become active in developing oral health education for the office and each patient. Community organizations generally look to local practices for dental health information or presentations for their patrons or employees. This is a good chance to become involved with other professionals in providing such education to those organizations. As a professional this is another duty or opportunity that can reap many rewards, both tangible and intangible.

Preparing a Lesson Plan for Specific Groups

In Chapter 5 you learned of the many different styles and levels of learning from prenatal to adolescents, and Chapter 6 discussed the styles and levels of adults. When designing a lesson plan, the educator will want to keep these styles and learning levels in mind. Using a template to develop lesson plans for any group helps keep the educator on track with the subject matter. It also assists in outlining the scope of the topic. Many dental professionals can discuss several aspects of oral health with great enthusiasm, yet their audience may have difficulty following the discussion if the professional goes off on a tangent subject. Outlining the lesson will ensure that the subject matter is well covered, and can allow for anecdotes and examples so the audience better comprehends the topic.

What is required in a lesson plan? Educators from preschool to postgraduate programs will develop some kind of lesson plan that allows them to effectively discuss a topic or event. Madeline Hunter (1982) developed the methodology of planning and presenting a lesson. Dr. Hunter surmised that no matter what the educator's style of teaching might be, the lesson could be designed as such that the students would gain knowledge. Success of the lesson then came in the form of measurements, otherwise known as tests. Measurements are based on the objectives in the lesson plan designed to "get the message across" using a variety of methods.

Essentially, the lesson plan has a goal, and the lesson is built around obtaining that particular goal. For example, when the dental hygienist begins patient education on flossing, what is the goal? Is the goal to get the patient *to* floss, or is the goal to get them understanding *why* they need to floss? By determining the goal, the dental hygienist can educate the patient more effectively. There are other steps in the lesson that assist the educator in measuring the success of the lesson. Table 9.2 lists the steps the educator can include when building a lesson plan based on Dr. Hunter's research.

As a student in dental hygiene school or a licensed practitioner, when looking at Table 9-2, it is obvious how chairside education with patients uses much of the format. Yet, you may not have been aware of how much of the oral health lesson actually followed a lesson plan model.

Now that there is better understanding of how a lesson plan is modeled, let's continue using the model and design a lesson for fluoride for a fourth-grade class. Remember in Chapter 5 that the development level for fourth-graders might include:

- Increased self-motivation
- Increased responsibility
- Increased ability to accept criticism and understand fairness
- May be enthusiastic about their own ideas
- Increased physical energy
- Increased need for change and variety versus routine tasks

TABLE 9.2 Lesson Plan Design

Anticipatory Set (focus)	A short activity or prompt that focuses the students' attention before the actual lesson begins. This is used when students enter the room or during a transition period between two subjects.
Purpose (objective)	The purpose of today's lesson, why the students need to learn it, what they will be able to do, and how they will show that they are learning as a result.
Input	The vocabulary, skills, and concepts the teacher will impart to the students. What it will take to be a successful student.
Modeling (show)	The teacher shows a graphic form or demonstrates what the finished product will look like.
Guided Practice (follow me)	The teacher leads the students through the steps necessary to perform the skill.
Checking for Understanding	The teacher uses a question-and-answer strategy format. For example: "Does everyone get the idea?" This also can set the pace of the lesson.
Independent Practice	The teacher releases students to practice on their own.
Closure	A review or recap of the lesson. The teacher may ask the students to repeat certain points of the lesson.

With these developmental changes occurring in the children, the lesson plan for fluoride might look similar to the following:

- **Anticipatory Set (focus):** Today's lesson will focus on fluoride. Where it is found, why it is important to our teeth, and how it is used. *(The educator may have some sample products that contain fluoride, which may pique the students' interest.)*
- **Purpose (objective):** After today's lesson the student will be able to: identify sources of fluoride, explain how fluoride works on teeth, discuss the importance of fluoride.

*The underlined terms are measurable objectives. When the student can perform these tasks with little or no assistance from the teacher, the student has gained knowledge of the subject.

- **Input:** Terms may include: fluoride rinses, teeth, protection, benefits, products
- **Modeling (show):** Have products that contain fluoride and use them to rinse as a demonstration to the students. Visual aids: a tooth model
- **Guided Practice (follow me):** Have the students follow rinsing or brushing. Provide verbal guidance while walking around the classroom assisting the students in their technique.
- **Checking for Understanding:** Ask feedback questions—"Where can you find fluoride?", "What does fluoride do to teeth?"
- **Independent Practice:** Homework handout—"Finding fluoride in my house"
- **Closure:** Ask the students what they have learned, and have them make a list on the chalkboard.

This lesson plan provides a variety of learning/teaching styles. There is some lecture, some individual tasks, and some interactive opportunities to keep the children interested and participating in the lesson. By incorporating a variety of settings for any lesson, the educator can be effective and successful with any subject matter. Additionally, by taking the time to understand the stages of development and learning styles for any age group, the lesson can be planned easily.

How to Teach to Specific Groups

Now that the lesson plan has been explained and demonstrated, how can this be used when targeting oral health to specific age levels or groups? Keeping in mind the material from Chapters 5 and 6, the oral health educator can identify criteria that will assist in the lesson plan development. Included with each lesson plan will be appropriate visual aids. Remember that those learning may be auditory or visual learners. When the dental health professional teaches oral health, the terminology can be overwhelming to the average consumer. Without the use of visual aids, the student-group may have difficulty in understanding what may be second nature to the oral health educator.

- **Preschool children.** This age group generally includes children from 2 to 5 years old. As discussed in Chapter 5, they are sensory learners. They want to touch, taste, smell, see, and hear everything around them. Teaching this group presents its challenges by way of keeping them interested enough that their attention is not diverted to something more exciting in the other part of the room. The lesson plans developed may include items that can be passed around as it is described by the teacher. Giving each child a toothbrush while explaining the bristles can allow the children to touch the bristles and place them against their teeth. Using toothpaste and allowing them to taste it may help them remember what toothpaste does for their teeth.

  As the oral health educator develops a lesson plan for preschoolers, it will be essential to incorporate "sensory" factors in hopes of keeping their attention and having them remember the important objectives of the lesson.

- **Elementary school–age children.** Children in this group will span from first-graders to sixth-graders. As they age, they become more independent and self-sufficient as well as more accountable. Maturity levels are wide ranging between first and sixth grade, thus lesson plans will want to incorporate tasks and information appropriate for the maturity level. For example, tobacco use may be more appropriate for fifth-graders versus first-graders. Although many oral health educators are aware that too many children are exposed to secondhand smoke should their parents be smokers, the information on tobacco use is more complex in nature, and those at a fifth-grade learning level are more apt to understand the consequences of tobacco use versus the first-grader. Likewise, the educator must be cautious to avoid "talking down" to a sixth-grade class. Using terminology that is appropriate to the age of the group or child helps in the comprehension of the lesson. During elementary school, children learn that teachers and parents have certain expectations in school and at home. When designing an oral health presentation, identifying expectations may assist the children in realizing that they may need to prepare themselves for answering questions as the presentation moves forward.

  Elementary school–age children are also more aware and skilled in the use of computers, not only for homework assignments but also for recreational use. Technology and home computers are not new to them, thus the health presentation may include technology in some way. Maintaining interest is also a challenge with any elementary level group. Interactive teaching methods will most certainly be an asset to presenting the lesson planned.

- **Pregnant teens.** By identifying commonalities among those who may be included in this group, the educator can incorporate the appropriate materials into the lesson. This particular group may have the following commonalities:
  - Under 18 years yet over 14 years
  - Physical development/their own and that of the fetus
  - Incomplete education
  - Lack of parental support

- Lack of participation from partners
- Living at home with parents
- Lack of income
- Use of local or state assistance

These commonalities can be used to develop an oral health lesson plan. The oral health educator will want to be aware to maintain a nonjudgmental demeanor. Bringing important health information to a group such as this can be a positive and significant influence to the teen mother and the unborn child. There is no way of knowing how much the pregnant teen may already know about oral health and the link it has to the health of her and her baby. Although pregnant, teens mentality rarely changes. Their attention span may be limited and it will require interactive tasks to be built into the lesson plan. By incorporating interactive tasks, teens are likely to remember more of the lesson. Perhaps the dental educator may include a sharing activity that discusses the teen's dental history, or their plans for the teething process as their child grows.

Visual aids can play a major role in the oral health message. The oral health educator may show a short film or demonstration video. Using terminology that teens can relate to can assist in maintaining their interest. Remember, dental terminology can be difficult to understand without using common terms and visuals. Small groups may alleviate shyness and generate more discussion, and perhaps allow teens to display some leadership skills by assigning a facilitator to each group.

In developing a list of commonalities for this particular group and taking the time to develop a diverse lesson plan, the oral health educator is sure to plan a successful presentation.

- **Young mothers/parents.** Young parents can range in age from 18 to 23. Here again, this is a group that may have diverse backgrounds. The oral health professional may find those with little education and of low socioeconomic status, to those with higher education and moderate income. The diversity can be great, yet when addressing oral health to this age group, the educator must be aware of the commonalities in the group. By identifying the common ground among the participants, the oral health lesson can be planned appropriately. For example, if a group of young parents are struggling financially, it will enhance the lesson plan to include products and merchants that can fall within a limited family budget. Likewise, perhaps the young parent group is unaware of dental insurance plans available to them, or perhaps dental offices that specialize in young children. Young parents may be more familiar with dental terminology and more apt to comprehend the significance of the oral health presentation. New parents are also interested in the development of the child, as everything occurs for the first time. Visual aids will assist in developing and explaining the oral health topics. Allowing some time in the lesson for the young parent to share his or her experience will also augment the subject matter in the lesson. They will have a greater sense of personalization. Thus, teaching a group of young parents can turn into an interactive discussion session versus a lecture.
- **Adults.** Adult learners require more complexity in the lesson planning. Adult learners are bringing more life experience to the learning environment. They will also have diverse levels of education. Technology can assist in the dental health lesson by way of

using slides or developing a PowerPoint presentation. Visual aids that enhance the verbal portion of the lesson are essential to maintain interest and generate questions. Adults may prefer to do the reading, thus the educator must facilitate the questions and the discussion. Creating a lesson that includes several formats will help to avoid boredom or loss of attention among the adult group. As many adult presentations are in the format of seminars, providing a break in the session at planned intervals will allow time for participants to refresh themselves.

- **The elderly.** Presenting oral health education to older adults can occur in a variety of settings: extended care facilities, residential nursing homes, and senior centers. The physical and mental capacity of the group will need to be established as the dental health educator will likely be addressing topics such as cancer, chemotherapy, partial and complete dentures, and systemic conditions that affect oral health and vice versa. Elderly groups may have some hearing loss and limited vision from distance positions in the learning environment. The dental educator may choose to design a presentation that works with smaller groups for more hands-on or personal attention to their needs. Perhaps the lesson plan will be more effective by having more than one educator present.

All of the groups presented are only a small sample of what kinds of things must be considered when building an effective oral health lesson. It will be imperative for the dental professional to identify common areas of the target group so as to incorporate appropriate elements in the lesson plan that will be most effective for learning.

Wrapping Up and Measuring the Results

As with any learning/teaching process, educators may agree that maintaining interest among the students or participants can be challenging. With all lesson planning it will be important to include sections of the lesson where interaction of some kind occurs. It could be sharing experiences, creating small-group discussion of a particular subject and presenting the results, or having the participants create an item that can be used in another lesson. No matter the type of interactive element, breaking up a pure lecture format is more likely to keep the group's interest.

Once the lesson is complete, having the group provide some feedback on the favorite section, least favorite section, or subject, allows them to reinforce what was presented. The educator then has the opportunity to check for understanding of the subject matter and clarify if necessary. One reason for measuring the results of the lesson is to find out whether or not the material in the lesson is effective, and what or how much the participants are retaining. Measuring the results of the lesson can be done on many forms: written quizzes, tests, question and answer, surveys, or evaluations.

In a classroom setting, quizzes and tests may be more appropriate. If the dental educator has presented a lesson in a community setting, an evaluation may be more appropriate. When using any measuring tool to identify the effectiveness of the lesson, the educator can design questions that focus on the objectives of the lesson plan. For example, if an evaluation form used in a community setting was designed on the fluoride lesson plan presented earlier, it might appear like the following:

Course Evaluation

Using the scale provided, please evaluate the course presented.

5 = Excellent   4 = Good   3 = Fair   2 = Satisfactory
1 = Needs improvement   NA = Not applicable

1. The objectives of the course were clearly stated.   5 4 3 2 1 NA
2. The objectives of the course met my needs.   5 4 3 2 1 NA
3. The topic was easy to understand.   5 4 3 2 1 NA
4. The visual aids enhanced the understanding of the material. 5 4 3 2 1 NA
5. The hands-on section enhanced the speakers' lecture.   5 4 3 2 1 NA
6. The audience had appropriate time for questions.   5 4 3 2 1 NA
Comments:

By using a measuring tool such as this evaluation, the educator can modify aspects of the lesson as suggested by participants. For any lesson, the dental professional will want to plan time for evaluation and modification. This allows for continued improvement and builds toward more concise and significant oral health presentations.

No matter what type of educational setting, whether it's chairside or a lecture hall filled with colleagues, building more effective lessons will augment and enhance the teaching style of the educator and the learning environment for those who participate.

Summary

As a dental professional it is essential to participate and understand the importance of standard of care for health care procedures. There is a shared responsibility among all licensed professionals in the way of patient care, consumer education, and ethics.

Realizing that all consumers have a basic need for safety and standard of care is a duty undertaken by health care professionals as they complete their education and become a member in the professional arena, a code of ethics has been established in dental hygiene and is upheld by those practicing in their respective field. Consumers expect that all health care professionals maintain their licensure by continued education and networking among colleagues.

Lesson plan development will require specific elements. These elements assist the dental educator in including appropriate subject matter and visual aids that will enhance the topic to the target group. It will also assist in allowing the inclusion of interactive teaching styles to maintain the interest and attention of the participants.

Teaching to specific groups will require the educator to identify common areas shared by members of the group. This will allow for personalization of the subject matter and creating an environment for participation from the audience members. Technology and creative visual aids will want to include a measuring tool for evaluating the oral health presentation. This is essential for continuous improvement in the presentations of the topic, the presentation styles, and the learning environment no matter the type of target group.

 # Critical Thinking

1. Select three of the basic human needs listed in the chapter and explain how they may present themselves in a clinical situation. For example, how would a need for a balanced diet apply to a patient seen in a dental office?
2. Briefly explain what is meant by the standards of care.
3. Explain the advantages for lesson plan development.
4. List the elements that are included in lesson planning.
5. Identify some common areas that may be shared by a group of pregnant teens.

 # Activities

1. Break into small groups and create a lesson plan on plaque prevention for a specific target group.
2. Create three visual aids for the caries process for a group of preschool children.
3. Class project: Develop a brochure on oral health and heart disease for adults.
4. Create a poster on oral piercing for high school–age teens.
5. Design a measurement tool for the lesson plan developed in question 1 above.

 # References

Darby, M. L., and M. M. Walsh. *Dental Hygiene Theory and Practice*. Philadelphia: W. B. Saunders, 1995.

Hunter, M. C. *Mastery Teaching*. Newbury Park, CA: Sage, 1982.

Kimbrough, V. J., and C. J. Lautar. *Ethics and Practice Management in Dental Hygiene*. New Jersey: Prentice Hall, 2003.

10

Partnering with Allied Health Practitioners and Educators

Objectives

Upon reading the material in this chapter, you will be able to

1. List resources in a community that will assist in advancing oral health education.
2. Discuss and outline goals on how others can teach dental health education.
3. Discuss steps to becoming a consumer advocate for improved oral health.
4. Discuss the benefits for membership in professional organizations.
5. Outline advantages for developing corporate partnerships.

Introduction

As a health care professional residing and working in any community, there will be an opportunity to become involved in the promotion of health and oral health education. By doing so, any health-oriented career can be more diverse, rewarding, and fulfilling. In each community, providing oral health education requires the work of many if the message is to be effective. The dental hygienist can play a major role as an advocate for consumers. Recognizing the many resources available will be key to getting others to share your vision and mission. Involving other health care providers will assist in getting the message out to everyone in the community by using various avenues for communication. There are numerous benefits to realizing that there are many agencies both public and private that can be approached as partners in developing and implementing a community health event of any nature.

How to Use Community Resources

Before anyone can use a community resource for any type of health program being designed, they must discover what kinds of resources are available to them. Many health professionals are aware that their community has agencies such as medical facilities, government agencies like the county health department, and agencies or businesses in the private sector. All of these entities will have a department or person that may be assigned to community events, public relations, or activities. Organizations that participate in community health projects can be found at the national, state, regional, and local levels. For example, the U.S. Department of Health and Human Services has a sector called the Health Resources and Services Administration (HRSA). HRSA's mission is to improve and expand access to quality health care for all. Health care is not exclusive to medical care; it includes oral health as well. HRSA is one of many agencies available as a resource for community health projects. Resources may include funding, educational materials, and workforce resources. HRSA attempts to address many areas affecting health in women, children, people with special needs, and rural populations. (See http://www.hrsa.gov.)

The next step will be to find out what private and public agencies are available in the state you may reside. Locating community resources can be as easy as browsing the Internet. Almost all public and private organizations have a website containing contact information along with information for both the consumer and the health professional.

Then many states or regions will have public health departments that focus on their immediate area with regard to all kinds of health concerns. For example, each state in the United States has counties, and each county has a health department. For other countries such as Canada, each province may have a public health agency designated for their province, region, or cities.

Next there is the private sector. Many organizations have a *foundation* or perhaps are philanthropic. Foundations and philanthropic organizations will also have vision and mission statements along with ongoing projects focused on improving health in their respective areas. These agencies tend to provide grant funding for large, health-focused projects that are likely to provide care, workforce resources, and supplies to professionals reaching out to rural areas, socioeconomically challenged consumers, or a special needs population. Many of these foundations work closely with higher education institutions and public health facilities. (Visit the Kansas Health Foundation website at http://www.kansashealth.org.)

The point is that all health and dental health professionals can become aware of the resources available to them as they become involved with designing and implementing community oral health education projects. By knowing where the resources are, the dental professional has the opportunity to expand a project, fund a project, and allow others to participate as partners in oral health education or services.

So how can dental health professionals use community resources? Most often, dental hygiene societies at both the state and local levels will decide to commit to and participate in an oral health project that selects a specific target group, such as children, or a specific dental health disease, such as caries. A project such as this requires a lot of planning to address areas like workforce, funding, supplies, transportation, public relations, and so many other things. Because there are so many factors to consider when planning an oral health project, the organizers will have to determine what they need from outside resources that also work with consumer health. For example, in 1994 the Washington Dental Service Foundation, along with Delta Dental, implemented a program called ABCD. It is active in 21 counties throughout Washington and focuses on preventive and restorative dental care for Medicaid-eligible children from birth to age 6. The program also advocates dental visits to begin as early as age 1 in order to address the caries process resulting in a lesser need for costly dental restorative work (http://www.abcd-dental.org). In order to create and employ this large project, it took the cooperation and resources of several partners and/or agencies, not to mention the many dental professionals who provided the education and performed the services. One of Washington's other outreach programs, titled "Cavity Free Kids," reached more than 16,000 children, awarded more than $1.5 million in grants and program support, and trained more than 7,500 individuals from 1998 to 2001 (Washington Dental Service Foundation, 2002). Statistics on oral health deficits, presented earlier in the text, indicates that nearly every community could benefit from this kind of oral health project.

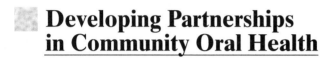

Developing Partnerships in Community Oral Health

The first step to designing a community project will be to assess and plan it (Figure 10.1).

In order for any community project to be successful, the development of partnerships will be a key factor. Let's look at the role each step plays in developing partnerships while designing a project or program that improves oral health.

STEP 1

The advisory committee: This committee works best when members are employed in diverse disciplines throughout the community. Additionally, when they are employed by health organizations or are business owners whose role is health-related, they are likely to take greater interest in the goals of the project and commit to participation.

STEP 2

Self-assessment and goals: This is where the advisory committee can determine the goals of the project, how long the project will run, and what resources are available to obtain the established goals.

STEP 3

The needs assessment: As the advisory committee continues to gain resources, assessing the needs of the target population based on the established goals will require some time and planning. Specific assignments can be given to the participants so that the task at hand is accomplished. As shown in Figure 10.2, this aspect of the project is large and the workforce assignments will require more detailed planning.

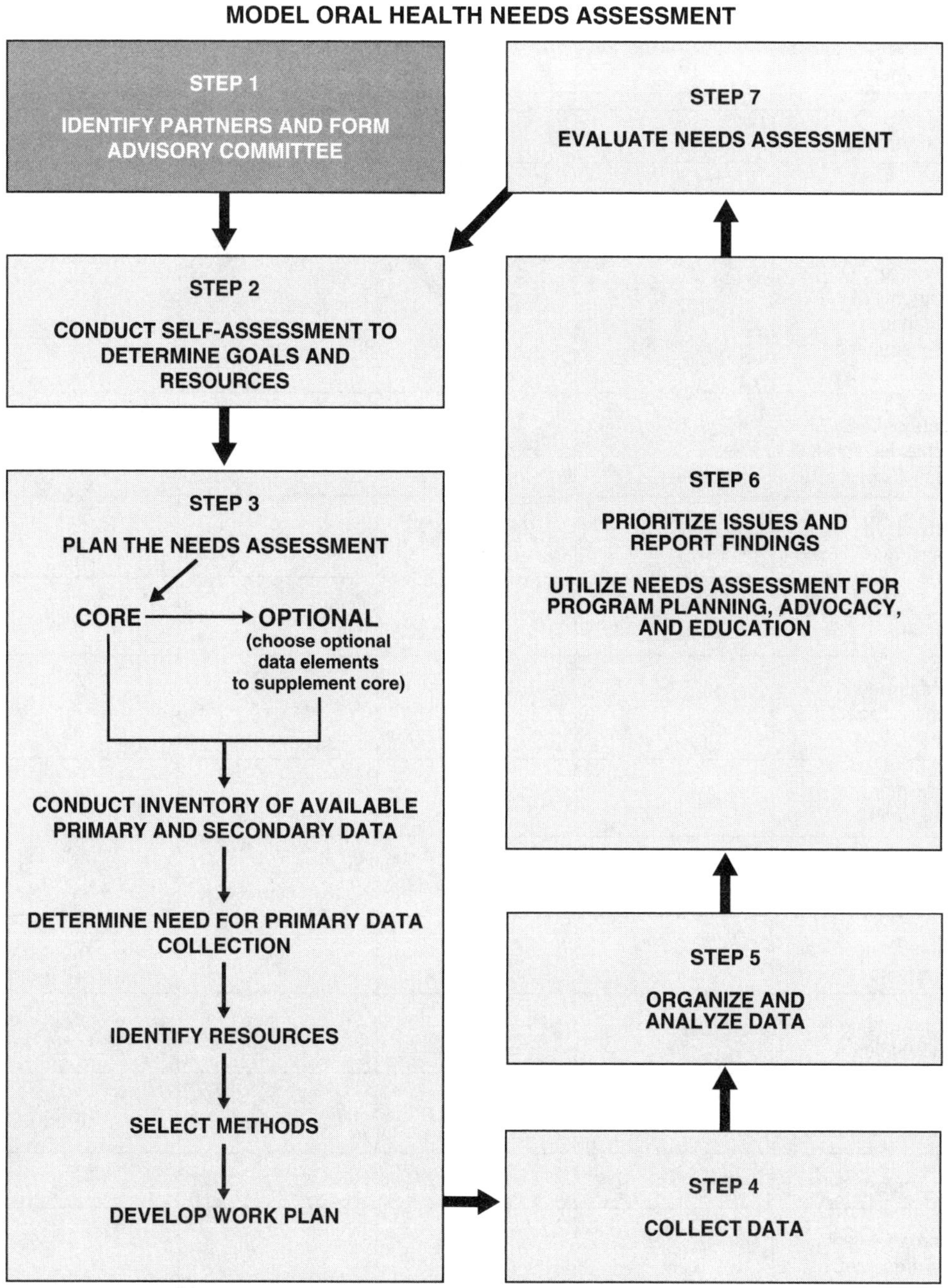

MODEL ORAL HEALTH NEEDS ASSESSMENT

STEP 1

IDENTIFY PARTNERS AND FORM ADVISORY COMMITTEE

STEP 7

EVALUATE NEEDS ASSESSMENT

STEP 2

CONDUCT SELF-ASSESSMENT TO DETERMINE GOALS AND RESOURCES

STEP 3

PLAN THE NEEDS ASSESSMENT

CORE ⟶ OPTIONAL
(choose optional data elements to supplement core)

CONDUCT INVENTORY OF AVAILABLE PRIMARY AND SECONDARY DATA

DETERMINE NEED FOR PRIMARY DATA COLLECTION

IDENTIFY RESOURCES

SELECT METHODS

DEVELOP WORK PLAN

STEP 6

PRIORITIZE ISSUES AND REPORT FINDINGS

UTILIZE NEEDS ASSESSMENT FOR PROGRAM PLANNING, ADVOCACY, AND EDUCATION

STEP 5

ORGANIZE AND ANALYZE DATA

STEP 4

COLLECT DATA

FIGURE 10.1 Seven-step model for assessing oral health needs and project planning. (*Source:* Association of State and Territorial Dental Directors, 1997)

Potential organizations and agencies	Advisory committee (Y/N)	Person	E-mail address	Telephone/fax
Oral Health				
State or Local Dental Association				
American Academy of Pediatric Dentistry, state chapter				
State or Local Dental Hygienists' Association				
Schools of Denistry				
Schools of Dental Hygiene				
Other: mental health, corrections, tribal				
Education Programs				
School of Public Health, Policy				
Other State/Local Programs				
Maternal and Child Health				
Children w/ Special Needs				
Medicaid/SCHIP				
Woman, Infants, Children (WIC)				
Epidemiology				

FIGURE 10.2 Sample worksheet—Forming an advisory committee. (*Source:* ASTDD Seven Step Model)

STEP 4

Data collection: Each project will require specific data in order to determine the needs as well as determine the success of the project based on the goals. Every project may have specific data forms that are custom designed, or perhaps available through the public health agencies that are partnered in the project.

STEP 5

Once collected, the statistics must be documented for baseline data, and compared to data collected at the end of the project. These statistics are often required for funding, and assist public health agencies in determining the needs of the community and/or the health of the community. It also provides information on how many consumers benefited from the project.

STEP 6

Prioritizing and reporting: Although any community health project will list many needs, there are some that will be more important than others. Most projects will look at the one thing that can benefit the majority for the longest time. For example, dental education and sealants may rank higher on the priority list than a dental visit. The partners for continued funding and overall evaluation of the project's operations generally require reporting outcomes of the project, its successes, and perhaps failures.

STEP 7

Evaluating the needs assessment: All projects, no matter the focus, must be evaluated. For those who have participated in a project, whether in the community or perhaps in your classroom, after implementing the plan, it becomes more apparent what areas require modification, enhancement, or elimination. Many projects appear good on paper, yet may not work as expected once begun. Evaluation is essential for continued improvement and success.

Now that there is a model to follow when planning a community project, where are the resources to contact? Table 10.1 lists some resources to consider when designing a community project.

As shown, any one of these organizations or agencies can be approached as a partner in promoting oral health. Creating an advisory committee with people from other disciplines enhances the opportunity to educate the community through many avenues and develop lasting partnerships with key players that share a similar vision.

These are but a few things to consider when designing an oral health program or project. There are many more details that will arise during the planning stage. Once the project is planned and outlined, those administrating the program can meet with numerous health agencies to assist with their project. Assistance will come in many forms, yet community leaders and health professionals continually work together to improve the quality of life for those in need. Community oral health projects require commitment and perseverance. The need is present, the desire to make a difference exists in many dental health professionals, and the community resources are available for many projects. Figure 10.2 is a sample worksheet to use as a guideline when designing a community outreach project that will involve partnerships.

For more sample worksheets, visit the website of the Association of State and Territorial Dental Directors at http://www.astdd.org.

TABLE 10.1 Oral Health and Health Resources That Can be Found in Many Communities

Dental Community:	*Medical Community:*
Private Practices	Private Practices
Local, State, and National Dental Societies	Specialty Practices
Local, State, and National Dental Hygiene Societies	Nurse Practitioners
Public Health Dental Clinics	Hospitals
Corporations: Dental Product Manufacturers	Long-Term Care Facilities
	Rehabilitation Facilities
Public Health:	*Private Sector:*
Health Departments	Health Foundations
State/Regional Aid Agencies	Residential Care Facilities
Family Service Agencies	Elderly Care Agencies
Social Service Agencies	Business Owners- Rotary Clubs, Lions Clubs
	Local Sports Clubs for Children/Adults

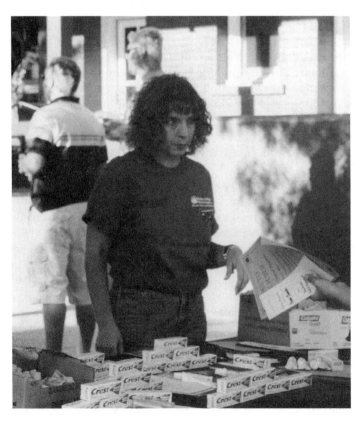

FIGURE 10.3 Dental hygiene student participating in a community event.

Teaching Others to Teach Oral Health Education

When becoming involved in a community project, whether large or small, it will be advantageous to enlist others to assist in oral health education. As a dental hygiene student your education was extensive in order to bring accurate information on oral health to your patients in order to motivate them to improve current habits. In a community setting, the basics of oral health will make all the difference in the world for those being reached. For example, many families may not have enough toothbrushes for every member. It is not a pleasant thought, however, it occurs more often that we care to admit. So, if a toothbrush can be provided to every person targeted by the project, the difference will be that each person now has the opportunity to begin being responsible for his or her own oral health.

In any outreach project, all participants or volunteer educators will need to learn basic oral health care and etiology of plaque and decay so that the community being targeted will gain more education from all project participants versus only a handful, which may be the dental professionals. When a dental professional teaches oral health care to a nondental person, terminology can be tricky, thus keeping it simple will result in better comprehension and communication. Table 10.2 provides some guidelines on the basics of oral health that the dental professional can focus on when educating a nondental professional, or another volunteer for a community outreach project.

As shown, when the dental professional provides basic information at a learning level for nondental professionals, there will be plenty to teach others. Focusing on these basic topics can assist in major improvements in oral health among all communities and target groups. Even though these topics are considered basic, as a dental hygiene student you know that there is a plethora of information that can be provided. However, keep in mind that too much information can cloud the main point: better oral health. When teaching an-

TABLE 10.2 Basic Oral Health Topics

Topic	Etiology/cause	Prevention
Plaque	Associated bacteria	Tooth brushing, flossing, diet
Decay	Plaque and acids	Tooth brushing, flossing, diet
Gum disease	Inflammation, infection, bleeding	Tooth brushing, flossing, diet, regular dental visits
Bone loss	Associated bacteria, disease progression	Tooth brushing, flossing, diet, regular dental visits
Calculus/tartar	Plaque associated, progression	Tooth brushing, flossing, dental visits
	Types	**Technique**
Tooth brushing	Power, manual, soft, sizes	Appropriate for dexterity and age
Flossing	Waxed, unwaxed, teflon	Properly demonstrated
Fluoride	Systemic, topical, rinse, drops/tablets, water	Professionally applied, home use

other person to teach oral health, staying on track with simple information will address the intent of the community project. It is similar to teaching chairside oral health with patients.

In an earlier chapter you learned that people have different ways of learning any subject matter. As it is likely those being taught to teach oral health in a community project are adults, the dental hygienist can use some of the teaching modalities discussed. For example, role-playing in teams will allow nondental community oral health educators to have the opportunity for critiquing each other's lesson plans. Prioritizing the main points for each oral health topic can help to streamline the message needing to be sent to those on the receiving end of the lesson. As community outreach projects will target people of all ages, it will be important to have appropriate visual aids, handouts, and educational materials that can be given as a reminder of the topics and education provided to the consumers. And because many projects are large in magnitude attempting to reach as many people as possible in a short amount of time, or in only one visit per year—keep the ultimate goal in mind: improved oral health. By educating all those involved as the workforce in a community project, all will share in the success and outcomes of the project.

Becoming a Consumer Advocate

Many seasoned dental hygienists find after spending many years in the clinical setting they have a desire to begin making a difference in their community as a consumer advocate. This means that they have a desire to assist members of the general public, low-income families, or elderly persons in changing or adding programs that target these populations. As a consumer advocate it will be essential to become aware of and stay informed on legal issues that may affect the population for which you are advocating. Legal issues may include health care, civil rights, labor, and employment.

On the state and national levels, legal issues occur daily and information is released to the public in large quantities. Legislation changes all the time due to budgetary constraints, a change in political leaders, and an increasing number of consumers who fall in any given category. The consumer advocate is likely to become a political figure within an organization or community. They strongly believe in change for the betterment of all consumers and are willing to challenge discriminatory and/or unfair laws and practices.

Consumer advocates are typically specialists in their field, such as a dental hygienist who has been in the workforce for several years and gained hands-on experience at the issues facing low-income families, diverse cultural groups, children, and older adults. It is possible that they have witnessed unfair practices targeting specific groups as those mentioned. Thus, they decide to change career directions and focus on changing how legislation addresses these target populations.

Since many issues facing specific consumer groups are of a legal nature, oftentimes the consumer advocate becomes involved with organizations that enlist the expertise of lawyers and other professionals more knowledgeable in areas that affect these groups. As a consumer advocate, access to such expertise is essential. Less often will a career dental hygienist run for elected office at the local level, or higher. However, there have been those who have been elected to their state legislative offices, and continue to change problem areas for many consumer groups and expand the practice of dental hygiene in their state.

As a dental hygienist, it is important to view the career as diverse in nature, and observe the many opportunities available to an oral health provider. Obtaining higher education and participating at all levels in the profession itself will enhance careers and open doors that never may have been thought of upon entering dental hygiene education.

As a consumer advocate, one has the opportunity to make significant changes in health care and other issues that face many specific target groups to ensure better overall health for everyone.

Professional Associations

As a dental hygiene student, your program may have asked you to become a member of the Student American Dental Hygienist's Association (SADHA). By doing so, this allows students to become involved with students from other programs at the local, state, and national levels as well as begin networking with the leaders of their associations. It also allows students to receive important professional journals that begin to enhance their career and advocate the scope of the dental hygiene profession.

More often, there are many licensed dental hygienists who have chosen not to become a member of their professional association, as they are unable to see the benefits associated with membership. As a member of any organization, members need to have something tangible to justify the annual membership fee. Tangibles will include items like medical insurance, malpractice coverage, and discount offerings. Oftentimes, intangibles outweigh tangibles and membership becomes a personal choice. Intangibles are items such as the opportunity to network with colleagues in other parts of the country, the opportunity to become a leader, and having a parent organization advocate for legislation at state and national levels.

Compare membership in the medical and dental profession to those in the dental hygiene profession. When a consumer seeks advice or consultation from a physician or dentist, they observe the many degrees and membership plaques that hang in his or her practice. What might the perception of the consumer be when observing these items? If you are the consumer, what perception do you have when you read that your physician or dentist has joined or participated in numerous professional organizations? What does the consumer think about the doctor or dentist who advertises the fact that they are a *fellow* in one organization, and a member in many others? Perhaps to the consumer this signifies that the doctor or dentist continues to network with colleagues and stay current on cutting-edge treatment modalities and medications. To the consumer, this might mean they will get higher quality treatment or service. This perception happens all the time. As a licensed health care professional and dental hygienist, membership in your professional association should mean nothing less than it would for the physician or the dentist. The patient in your chair perceives that membership in a similar manner as that of the dentist or physician. As an oral health care professional, the consumers are owed the highest quality of care, and a provider that holds the highest standards of ethics. When the consumer knows that their care provider is a member of their professional association, they believe that the dental hygienist remains current on cutting-edge treatment and products. From the consumer's standpoint the dental hygienist is just as important as the dentist or the physician. All dental hygienists owe it to their patients to take part in all aspects of their profession.

Professional associations are an excellent resource for each member and for consumers. Many of them have websites that include a consumer page, and a professional page filled with educational information, legal issues facing consumers and professionals at the national level, press releases, and research materials. Many also provide funding for education and community projects that are focused on improving oral health. (Visit the American Dental Hygienists Association website at http://www.adha.org.)

Professional associations are advocates for both consumers and licensed professionals. As the scope of dental hygiene practice changes from state to state, allowing increased access to care, and promoting oral health and education, it will be essential for all licensed professionals to actively participate in their professional organizations and communities.

Summary

Communities face increasing numbers of consumers that require oral health and education in nontraditional settings. Creating outreach projects will provide access to education and services. These outreach projects take planning and funding that require participants from all aspects of any community. The dental hygienist can play a key role within an organization or as the leader in designing an outreach project. By creating an advisory committee that shares the same vision and mission for improved oral health, the resources for funding, materials, and a workforce can be identified and planning can proceed smoothly. Recognizing corporate partnerships and establishing a link will augment any community project and include others dedicated to improving health in their community. Partnerships can assist in establishing goals and achieving success in the project.

All those participating in a community project can be taught to provide oral health education. Identifying the basics of oral health and what is needed to prevent disease will allow the dental educator to focus on priorities for such education in a community setting. Keeping it simple to ensure comprehension by those who must learn to teach oral health will make it much easier to get the message to this highest number of consumers targeted by the outreach project.

The dental hygienist can often enhance his or her career by becoming a consumer advocate and working on health issues that face specific populations in their community. Many often leave the clinical setting to become legislative leaders working for consumers and their profession.

Professional associations are not only designed to service licensed professionals, they are also designed to be accessible to consumers. Many publish and release consumer educational materials, as well as servicing the professional with benefits and research material. Consumers perceive any health professional as being on the cutting edge of new treatment modalities when membership in their respective professional association is secured. All licensed dental hygienists have a responsibility to themselves as well as their patients to hold membership in their professional association.

 # Critical Thinking

1. When designing a community outreach project, what is the purpose for establishing an advisory committee?
2. Why is it important to perform a needs assessment prior to a community health project?
3. When collecting data from a needs assessment or community dental health survey, what information might it give to community health professionals?
4. What role might a consumer advocate play in an oral health advisory committee?
5. Perceptions of consumers can be difficult to change. Many consumers do not believe that visiting their dental professional on a regular basis is necessary. As a dental hygienist, what are some ways to change the consumer perception on the importance of regular preventive dental care?
6. Group discussion: List the tangibles and intangible reasons for professional membership in the American Dental Hygienists' Association. Divide into two groups: one group are members, the other is not. Discuss your justifications for membership or nonmembership.

 # Activities

1. As a class, establish what might be an oral health need in the community. Once this has been agreed upon, use the worksheet in Figure 10.2 to establish participants for an advisory committee.
2. Identify local, state, and/or national organizations that may assist in the community project for question 1.
3. Form groups of four or five students. Select one student to be the oral health educator that must teach the others (nondental persons) on how to teach an oral health topic.
4. As a class, select an issue that faces a specific target population. For example, transportation to health appointments for geriatric consumers. Have one student volunteer to be a consumer advocate fighting to change the problems with transportation issues, while the other class members act as legislators who are either for or against the changes.

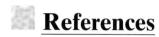 # References

Association of State and Territorial Dental Directors. *Assessing Oral Health Needs: ASTDD Seven Step Model 1997.* http://www.astdd.org.

Washington Dental Service Foundation. *Improving Community Oral Health, Cavity Free Kids, a Pilot Program.* http://www.deltadentalwa.com, 2002.

11

The Consumer's View
of Oral Health Products

Objectives

Upon reading the material in this chapter, you will be able to

1. Identify the benefits of fluoride in community water systems.
2. Discuss the position of fluoride use held by dental professional organizations.
3. Identify the benefits and uses for pit and fissure sealants.
4. Discuss the advantages for over-the-counter consumer oral health products.
5. Discuss the disadvantages of product media marketing from the consumer's perspective.

Introduction

During your tenure as a dental hygiene student, you likely had the opportunity to view television commercials of many dental products. Undoubtedly, as you became more knowledgeable about oral health and products, you also realized how marketing could affect the average consumer when it comes to certain products, such as tooth whitening. As more and more products become available to the consumer via their local supermarket or drug store, the consumer then becomes their own dental health professional and actively self-prescribes what will be the best product for their need.

This is something all dental health professionals will want to be aware of when assessing their patient in order to determine what products may be recommended as they improve their oral health status. As a dental hygienist, one of the goals for improved oral health in the patient is to get them to own their present oral health condition, and realize that they play an important role for improving that condition. The patient needs to realize that he or she is an important partner, and the dental professional can guide them to the most appropriate product that will assist in maintaining their oral health.

There are numerous products, both brandname and generic, that can cause the consumer to be perplexed and confused as they attempt to self-prescribe the product that will improve and maintain their oral health status. The dental hygienist can stay abreast and informed on dental care products that enter the market each year, so that they are recommending appropriate oral health aids for all of their patients. Although this text is not designed to cover all dental products available to the consumer, it is essential for the dental hygienist to realize what the consumer faces when selecting a dental product. Let's examine how the consumer might view some of these products and how the dental professional can lead them in the right direction.

Fluoride Products/Systems

There are consumers using fluoridated products without realizing the true benefits of fluoride. They use it because their dentist or dental hygienist told them to, yet perhaps do not explain why. Then there are consumers who specifically tell their dental hygienist they do not want fluoride in any of the products recommended. When challenged in multifaceted ways by the many patients seen each year, it will be the background knowledge the dental professional can bring to their patients to help them understand how certain product ingredients can enhance their oral health. Caution must be used when recommending all products containing fluoride because there are conditions that arise when too much eliminates the benefits sought from the agent, such as enamel fluorosis.

Pediatricians recommend for many new parents to use fluoride drops while the child is developing teeth, because the fluoride aids in a harder enamel structure prior to tooth eruption. However, there are specific limits of fluoride that must be adhered to prevent enamel fluorosis. Table 11.1 provides the recommended dosage of fluoride for children as developed and endorsed by the American Dental Association, the American Academy of Pediatrics, and the American Academy of Pediatric Dentistry.

As mentioned, fluoride can be a controversial topic for many consumers. However, for the majority of dental health professionals, it is a substance that has proven itself for decades in the prevention and decrease of caries through strengthening of the enamel

TABLE 11.1 Recommended Dosage of Fluoride by Age

Age	Fluoride ion level in drinking water (ppm)*		
	< 0.3 ppm	0.3–0.6 ppm	> 0.6 ppm
Birth to 6 months	None	None	None
6 mos–3 yrs	0.25 mg/day**	None	None
3–6 yrs	.50 mg/day	0.25 mg/day	None
6–16 yrs	1.0 mg/day	0.50 mg/day	None

* 1.0 ppm = 1 mg/liter
** 2.2 mg sodium fluoride contains 1 mg fluoride ion
Source: American Dental Association, 2004

structure. Dental hygienists look to fluoride for several reasons: decreased decay, decreased sensitivity, and increased mineralization of tooth surfaces. Consumers, dental hygiene students, and seasoned professionals are encouraged to visit the American Dental Association website for extensive information and facts on fluoride at http://www.ada.org. However, it is especially appropriate to establish some basic facts at this time.

From a scientific standpoint, the fluoride ion stems from *fluorine*, which exists as an element on earth in the same way oxygen exists. Believe it or not, fluorine is the 17th most abundant element in the earth's crust and only exists in combination with other elements as a fluoride compound (Largent, 1970). Fluoride ions result in nature as water erodes rock formations possessing fluoride compounds. Therefore, small amounts of fluoride can be found in all aspects of the earth, especially in water sources and oceans (National Academy of Sciences, 1977). As the world's population increases, the community water sources have varied concentrations of naturally occurring fluoride in most industrialized nations.

Since 1950, the ADA, along with the United States Public Health Services (USPHS), has continuously endorsed the fluoridation of community water supplies as the most effective way to decrease caries and caries risk. Adding fluoride, or rather adjusting the fluoride concentration, to a community water source allows an optimal level of fluoride to reach millions of consumers at very little cost. After extensive research by the USPHS, optimal community water fluoride concentration was established as a range of 0.7 to 1.2 parts per million. This means that one milligram per liter (mg/L) is equal to one part per million (ppm). Thus, at 1 ppm, one part of fluoride is diluted in a million parts of water. The range was established due to the fact that naturally occurring fluoride in water sources will be different in geographic areas of the earth. The range then allows a concentration of fluoride that has been deemed effective to reduce tooth decay, yet minimize the chance for *enamel fluorosis* (USDHHS-CDC, 1986). Fluorosis occurs when there is disruption in the tooth enamel during the mineralization process prior to eruption.

Many who oppose community water fluoridation may not be aware that its effectiveness has been documented in scientific literature since 1945, while fluorosis and its relation to dental caries can be researched back to 1938 in an article by H.T. Dean and published by Public Health Reports. Those in opposition state that fluoride is a toxic chemical and a carcinogen. There are many antifluoridation activist groups, and for a better understanding of antifluoridation an Internet search can be done using key words (go to any search engine and enter "antifluoridation" into the search window).

There are many ways to apply fluoride: topical—self-applied, topical—professionally applied, systemic through supplements, community water systems, or bottled water. When the dental hygienist is going to recommend home fluoride therapy it will be essential to educate the patient on how to use the product correctly. There are mouth rinses, concentrated rinses, brush-on gels, and more. When asking the patient to purchase a fluoride product for home care, the clinician will want to be specific on the type of product and how to use the product. Figure 11.1 shows the oral care product aisle that can be seen in any supermarket or drug store. The consumer is faced with a huge decision if the dental professional allows them to make that decision on his or her own with no guidance. Thus, there is the possibility that the patient gives up and purchases nothing—and compliance does not take place in between their dental hygiene visits.

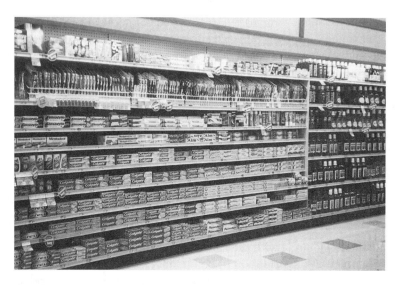

FIGURE 11.1 Supermarket aisle display of oral health products.

In summary, dental hygienists will be one of the first consumer contacts to provide their patient with knowledge on agents such as fluoride. Many will encounter patients that prefer to stay away from agents such as fluoride. Patient education will be the key to ensure that all patients are making informed decisions on any product or agent designed to improve oral health.

Toothbrushes

Toothbrushes have undergone major design changes over the last 10 years. In addition to the change in manual brushes, the increased technology for power brushes, once known as the electric brush, dictates that the dental hygienist stay current with what is being offered to the consumer. All of the major oral care product manufacturers rely on the dental professional to promote their product to consumers. These corporate entities are also increasing their professional personnel as they hire dental hygienists for their research and development departments, their education departments, and their sales departments. Let's face it, who knows better about the use of oral care products than the dental professional? Thus, dental manufacturers are increasingly savvy in how they promote themselves to becoming a common household name. The example of such marketing is indicated by the sales of oral hygiene products, reaching over $4 billion in 2000 (ADHA, 2004).

The dental hygienist understands the sole purpose of the toothbrush: to remove soft plaque deposits and food debris. Other benefits arise from the mechanical action of toothbrushing, such as gingival health, and decreased extrinsic stain. Yet with so many new brush designs, the consumer may have more questions as manufacturers target their media marketing to the general public.

Generally speaking, manual toothbrushes should have the following characteristics:

- Conforms to shape, size, and texture of the patient's preferences
- Easily and effectively manipulated around the mouth
- Can be cleaned and dried, with bristles that do not absorb moisture
- Durability and affordability
- Soft, flexible bristles and a rigid, lightweight handle
- Bristles that have rounded ends

Source: Wilkins, 2005

The dental professional will recommend a specific toothbrush for many reasons, all of which are listed above, yet also with keeping the patients' oral needs in mind as well as their physical ability to manipulate a manual brush. Selection of a toothbrush by the patient may not include the criteria listed above. Their view could be that all toothbrushes are the same, since they are all used in the same manner. The dental hygienist will want to educate the patient during their regular visits, so that whenever the patient is faced with the decision on a toothbrush, they are making a more informed decision that includes efficiency of the brush itself.

Electric toothbrushes have evolved into the power toothbrush. The early mechanics of the power brush simulated the motion of manual toothbrushing techniques. Presently, this motion has increased in speed as well as motions that cannot be duplicated by manual brushes (Wilkins, 2005). The overall purpose of the power toothbrush is the same: removal of soft deposits and food debris. One of the major benefits observed by practitioners is that gingival recession can be decreased because the patient who "scrubs" is not able to use the power brush in the same way they would maneuver a manual toothbrush. The design of the power toothbrush is something to consider when recommending one to patients. Here again, their oral needs will assist in that recommendation. Cost of the power toothbrush will be a deciding factor from the patient's standpoint. The average cost ranges from approximately $40 to $130 for a power brush. As a result, many manufacturers have designed a battery-operated version of a power toothbrush. This allows the consumer another choice when stepping up from a manual toothbrush.

Here again is another product line that presents numerous choices and benefits for the consumer. The dental hygienist can provide greater insight and information to their patient so that they are making well-informed decisions about oral health care and selecting the best product for their needs.

Dental Floss

Dental hygienists can tell many stories about the number of patients they see each year that refuse to use dental floss. Their reasons are many and may be quite creative, yet the practitioner realizes the need for flossing, and also realizes that they may never change the mind of many nonflossers. One of the reasons consumers don't like to floss is because it breaks when using it between posterior teeth and then are left with tiny strands of floss fibers. Along with technological improvements for toothbrushes, floss has also seen changes that allow the patient to manipulate it easier than before. This aids in addressing the nonflosser's justification that their fingers are too big.

Being a dental hygienist exposes many to new products through direct mail marketing as well as sales representatives. Many practitioners often participate in their state or national dental or dental hygiene conventions where all manufacturers display and educate the professionals on their wares. However, what does the consumer see? Dental floss comes in many forms: unwaxed, waxed, teflon, gortex, and more. In addition, it comes in many design types: flat, round, ribbon, tape, braided, and so on. Then there are the specialized versions: those impregnated with baking soda, antimicrobial agents, and fluoride. Of course, for those patients stating they cannot get their fingers in their mouth, there are the floss holders: designed for everyone in mind—including kids! Next, we can list the many flavors of floss. Manufacturers have done everything possible to gain acceptance by the average consumer no matter what their taste or preference. As a result of endless choices, the consumer may not have any idea where to begin.

The dental hygienist will want to recommend the appropriate product and educate the patient on characteristics to look for when shopping for dental floss. The consumer is challenged by the number of choices and will appreciate that the practitioner can provide the knowledge needed to select the right product. Dental floss recommendations are also based on the needs of the patient's oral condition, yet the challenge is to find one that is easy to manipulate so that the patient complies with their oral home care.

Mouthrinses

When standing in their local supermarket or drug store, the dental patient recalls that his or her dental hygienist has been recommended to rinse with a mouthrinse twice daily to reduce bacteria. All right, but which one? Does one work better than the other? Is one supposed to be the best? These may be but a few questions going through the patient's mind as they attempt to determine which rinse is best for them.

Generally, the United States Food and Drug Administration (FDA) have classified mouthrinses as either therapeutic or cosmetic. Some may be a combination of the two. Removing food debris, eliminated bad breath, and leaving a fresh taste are characteristics of the cosmetic rinse. Rinses designated as therapeutic will have some of the same characteristics yet will also include specific ingredients designed to protect against oral diseases such as gingivitis and caries. Therapeutic rinses are regulated by the FDA and voluntarily approved by the ADA (AGD, 2004).

The dental hygienist learns through education and exposure that some rinses are developed to decrease the risk of caries by the addition of fluoride and perhaps agents that will decrease bacteria. Other rinses may be more antiseptic and target bacteria that will cause caries and gingivitis. There are also prescription rinses containing chlorhexidine gluconate that assist in bacterial elimination during active periodontal diseases.

So what does the patient standing in front of mouthrinses select? Hopefully, the one his or her dental hygienist has recommended. The latest television advertisements are advocating that certain mouthrinses are "as effective as flossing." When the consumer views this kind of promotion, they may be hearing, "Eliminate your floss by using this rinse." What might this say to that nonflosser you've been working so diligently to convert? The dental practitioner will want to take the time to educate their patient and use caution when it comes to advertising oral care products. Clinicians are aware that using anything to remove debris and bacteria will be better than nothing. However, all products have their limits. There is no one single "miracle" cure or easy way out when it comes to improved oral health.

Tooth Whitening Systems

Yes, this is the area where many consumers are targeted by product manufacturers as well as the need for a whiter smile. Television marketing has increased in the last few years for whitening products, which began with whitening toothpastes. This marketing frenzy has now extended into whitening products that are closer to professional products found only in the dental practice yet only a fraction of the cost. The problem lies in that the consumer does not realize that not all teeth will whiten due to many factors, and the dental hygienist can be a great resource of information on whitening products.

Whitening toothpastes remain on the market, although they have improved with time. Consumers do not understand that most whitening toothpastes are designed to remove extrinsic or superficial stains, thus allowing the teeth to appear whiter. The consumer also does not realize that intrinsic or embedded stains such as tobacco or stains resulting from antibiotic therapy may not be removed with toothpaste alone. Additionally, they do not know that anterior restorations such as composites, crowns, and veneers will not be improved by whitening products. What they do know is what they see in advertisements—white teeth in 14 days!

What choices do consumers have when it comes to whitening products? There are many at-home products that the consumer can be directed toward. First is the at-home bleaching kit. This allows the dentist or dental hygienist to fabricate a custom tray for the patient and provide them with a whitening solution to place into the tray and wear for a specified period of time. The whitening gel solution is generally a carbamide peroxide concentration that can come in different strengths. Many clinicians observe increased temperature sensitivity with the higher concentrations, yet this effect dissipates once the whitening process is completed. Within a few weeks, the teeth have become significantly whiter.

Then there are the over-the-counter products such as Crest White Strips or Colgate Simply White, which the consumer can purchase in any drug store. The whitening solution may be at a lower concentration level for consumer safety, yet over time, teeth become whiter. The lasting effects of any product will vary.

Next there are power-whitening techniques. Lasers are not used anymore due to the possibility of tooth damage; a curing light activates a whitening gel product that accelerates the whitening process, and the final result is reached in about an hour or perhaps over a period of a few treatments. This cannot be done at home.

Tooth whitening products can be found via infomercials, yet many of these products could be generic in nature and dental professionals or reputable dental product manufacturers do not guarantee the efficacy and safety of these products.

As more and more patients request whiter teeth, their choices of how to obtain this are increasing. Here again, cost for such products and procedures will range widely. Over-the-counter products may begin as low as $15, yet the amount of time to get the desired result will take longer. Professional whitening can start as low as $100 and rise from there depending on the technique. The dental hygienist can aid in providing appropriate information on whitening products so that the consumer is making the best choice in product and procedure. Harm can be done with many products and the consumer is better protected when educated on aspects of oral care products.

 ## Pit and Fissure Sealants

During your dental hygiene education, you have come to understand the short-term and long-term benefits for sealant application, especially in children. However, many consumers fail to realize their benefit. Many view them as unnecessary because they are placed on "baby teeth, which are going to fall out anyway." Additionally, the cost of sealant placement per tooth ranges from dentist to dentist and from area to area. There are still dental insurance plans that do not include sealants, despite the fact they have been standard preventive recommendations in dentistry for over 20 years.

All dental practitioners know that sealants are designed to protect the tooth surface from decay-causing bacteria. When sealants are placed on younger children, it allows the child's manual dexterity to mature so that toothbrushing becomes more efficient with age. Meanwhile, the tooth has been protected from possible caries development.

Many parents have been slow to accept dental disease prevention. Dentistry in general has experienced this slow acceptance in those families that are economically challenged versus those who are not. Parents stemming from families where oral health stood low on the priority list are now facing the same decisions their parents faced when it comes to preventive care versus urgent care. The cycle seems to perpetuate in each generation.

One of the most difficult challenges for the dental hygienist is to reach parents and consumers of all ages and educate them on the advantages of oral health prevention. Sealant placement on appropriate tooth surfaces has been one of the key factors in preventive treatment. The general public will always view preventive care differently than the practitioner. The consumer has to balance many things for their families, and anything that is preventive is viewed as costly. Dental professionals know that urgent care is more costly than preventive care, yet are unable to change the viewpoints of their patients who are generally treated under urgent circumstances. By taking an active role in patient education on numerous levels, the dental hygienist can make a small difference that has the potential to grow. Educating all parents on why sealants are beneficial will assist the consumer in choosing preventive practices.

 ## The ADA Seal of Acceptance Program

Oftentimes patients will only want to use products that are ADA approved. For them, this means that the product is better than one that does not have "the seal." So what does this seal really mean, and why do some products have them and others do not?

The ADA's Seal program began in 1930 and was established to oversee the evaluation of dental products through the Council on Dental Therapeutics. The ADA Seal of Acceptance is a registered certification mark of the American Dental Association. Currently, this Council is now known as the Council on Scientific Affairs and is responsible for the dissemination of information regarding safety, efficacy, promotional claims, and proper use of dental therapeutic agents (ADA, 2004).

This process of obtaining a seal of approval is voluntary at the request of the manufacturer, distributor, or the Council. Products may be accepted on a provisional basis, which means that the Council does not have sufficient evidence or information to fully accept and approve the product.

Table 11.2 identifies some of the criteria required for the process for gaining the ADA Seal of Acceptance/Approval.

Often, when the dental hygienist is questioned by their patient on particular products, the patient will inquire as to whether or not the product is ADA approved. Understanding what it takes for any dental product to obtain the Seal of Acceptance can provide some

TABLE 11.2 Abbreviated Version of the Criteria for the Seal of Acceptance Program, Areas I–VI.

I. Names	Established or generic names must conform to FDA requirements and the Cosmetic Act. Trade names cannot be misleading or suggest diseases. "DDS" or "DMD" are not acceptable in the name of the product.
II. Composition, Nature, and Function	Product information and manufacturing standards must include the ingredients, composition, and properties, and be done in controlled facilities with qualified personnel. The company must provide evidence that the product demonstrates compliance with its guidelines or specifications.
III. Evidence of Safety and Efficacy	Evidence must be provided pertaining to the actions, safety, and efficacy regarding the mechanical and physical properties. Objective data from clinical and laboratory studies are submitted. Post marketing surveillance regarding safety and efficacy must be submitted when available.
IV. Government Regulations	Product must conform to government regulations.
V. Biodegradable/Recyclable Materials	ADA encourages all manufacturers to use biodegradable or recyclable materials whenever possible.
VI. Labeling, Package Inserts, Advertising	Name must be prominent/claims of significance to dentistry must be clear and accurate/all printed related material must be reviewed. Advertising must not disparage other products. Advertising must conform to ADA standards. Accepted products must not be displayed with unaccepted products that would imply the acceptance of the other products.

Source: American Dental Association, 2004

assurance of the quality of the product and the integrity of the product's manufacturer. Since the Seal program is voluntary, manufacturers are not likely to enter the process of the program without having confidence in their product and the benefits it can bring to consumers. The dental professional will also be able to have confidence in the products they are recommending for their patients.

Advertising Dental Products

Since this chapter attempts to point out the consumer's perspective on dental products, it is warranted to also point out how the marketing and advertising of these products send certain messages to the consumer. These messages are then brought to the dentist and dental hygienist as requests or questions by the patient, because they have essentially diagnosed themselves with the condition being depicted in the advertisements. For example, as mentioned earlier, there are television ads that have run in the fall of 2004 by a top-selling mouthrinse company indicating that by using their mouthrinse daily, "it is as effective as flossing." How does the patient receive this message? Perhaps they begin to think that a miracle rinse has been invented to purposefully eliminate the reasons to floss. How does the dental hygienist receive this message? Savvy dental professionals are well aware of the product ingredients and can reason that there will be a reduction in oral bacteria, yet will be a limited removal of debris. The message has been received in two very different manners.

Dental professionals are well aware of the battle between power toothbrush makers, each one indirectly (or perhaps directly) indicating they are better than the other when it comes to removing plaque and debris, so much better that oral diseases are decreased dramatically. How does the consumer view this type of marketing? Perhaps they receive the message that says, "your oral disease will never improve unless you are using this power toothbrush and no other."

Another example is when antimicrobial/antibiotic products came onto the scene in the 1990s. One antibiotic manufacturer released headlines that indicated periodontal disease could now be eliminated by taking the medication. The consumer received the message that went something like this, "Take this pill once each day and eliminate gum disease forever and never have to see your dental hygienist again." Sounds ridiculous, right? Being the educated dental hygienist, yes it does sound ridiculous. But to the consumer, it may mean their life just got easier.

Advertising and marketing of dental products is something that must occur for the success of any business. Advertising can sometimes mislead the average consumer by the way the message is stated or depicted. The dental hygienist has sufficient scientific education, as well as staying current on new technology, that the patient can be provided accurate information on any product available to them.

Whenever working with patients or perhaps the general public in a community environment, the best education the dental hygienist can provide will include the understanding of what is being presented to consumers by product manufacturers, advertising, and marketing. Presenting accurate information to all patients will assist them throughout their lifetime in selection of the oral care products that are best for them whatever their oral health may be.

Summary

Dental professionals and consumers view dental products and procedures differently. Many consumers do not realize that there is certain aspects of advertising and marketing that are designed to draw them in, yet certain products are not going to work well for everyone.

Fluoride holds numerous benefits for the dental hygienist. They have been educated on the scientific background of fluoride and have a better understanding as to why their patients, both young and old, will benefit from its use. Pediatricians recommend fluoride for infants due to its systemic benefit during the development of tooth enamel prior to eruption. Fluoride occurs naturally in all water sources on the earth. The majority of cities and nations do not have optimal fluoride levels in the drinking water that will aid in decreasing decay rates. Yet there are many who also oppose water fluoridation because they view it as a toxic substance.

Dental products such as toothbrushes, mouthrinses, and dental flosses are all changing as a result of technology. This technology has a positive impact on oral health in general. However, technology also brings increased costs to the consumer as well as numerous selections. The dental hygienist can be a great resource of information for their patients and assist in directing them to the appropriate choices for their oral condition as well as their lifestyle.

Pit and fissure sealants have been used in dentistry for well over 20 years, yet many parents still do not see the benefits for sealants on deciduous teeth, and some dental insurance companies have not included them as part of their preventive care. Continued education for parents will be key in accepting preventive measures in dental care.

Whitening products vary in cost and availability to the consumer, yet many do not realize the conditions for which they will be more successful. The "whiter" smile is something that more consumers are requesting, while preventive and restorative procedures may be lower priority. The dental practitioner will want to stay current on all products that may be accessible to their patients in supermarkets and drug stores so that the patient is directed to a safe and effective product.

Dental product manufacturers target the consumer on a daily basis. Oftentimes the messages sent by product manufacturers influence consumers to self-diagnose their oral condition and seek professional treatment based on their assessment. The message received by consumers as a result of advertising and marketing will be vastly different than the message received by the educated dental hygienist. The practitioner then has the opportunity to provide the patient with scientific background on the product and the properties in which it works.

Overall, patient education is key to successful improvement of total health and most importantly oral health. The dental hygienist is one of the best dental professionals to provide such important education.

Critical Thinking

1. As a class discuss community water fluoridation. Does your community fluoridate the water to an optimal level? What is the current level of fluoride in the water system? Is this a controversial issue in the community?

2. Share experiences that may have occurred during clinic sessions or private practices where a patient requested nonfluoridated agents.

3. Discuss the many designs of manual toothbrushes and dental floss available to consumers. Why might some of these items be confusing to the patient who has not been educated by the dental hygienist?

4. List some of the whitening products offered to consumers via television advertisements. Can you identify statements that may be misleading when heard by the consumer?

5. Discuss current television advertisements of dental products. What kind of messages are being sent? How might the consumer receive the message? As a dental hygiene student, how do you receive the message?

Activities

1. Research the Internet for antifluoridation positions. What claims are being made? Does the position being taken have scientific or clinical backing?

2. Visit a local supermarket or drug store and observe the many dental products available to the consumer. How many of the products have the ADA Seal?

3. Conduct an informal survey with patients, classmates, coworkers, family members, on their preference of floss. Which floss brand/type is most preferred and why?

4. In small groups, select a dental product and create an advertising campaign that will run during the month of October (National Dental Hygiene Month). What is your message to the consumer? Can you be assured the message is received as it is intended?

References

American Academy of General Dentistry. *What are the Differences in Rinses?* http:// www.agd.org, 2004.

American Dental Association. *Frequently Asked Questions, Fact Sheets, Position Statements.* http://www.ada.org, 2004.

American Dental Hygienists' Association. http://www.adha.org, 2004.

Dean, H. T. Endemic Fluorosis and Its Relation to Dental Caries. *Public Health Reports, 53* (33) (1938), 1443–1452.

Dean, H. T., F. A. Arnold, and E. Elvove. Domestic Water and Dental Caries. *Public Health Reports, 57* (32) (1942), 1155–1179.

U. S. Department of Health and Human Services, Centers for Disease Control, Dental Disease Prevention Activity. *Water Fluoridation: A Manual for Engineers and Technicians.* Atlanta, GA: Author, 1986.

Wilkins, E. M. *Clinical Practice of the Dental Hygienist,* 9th ed. Baltimore: Lippincott, Williams & Wilkins, 2005.

Appendix A

Dentition Eruption Tables

PRIMARY TEETH

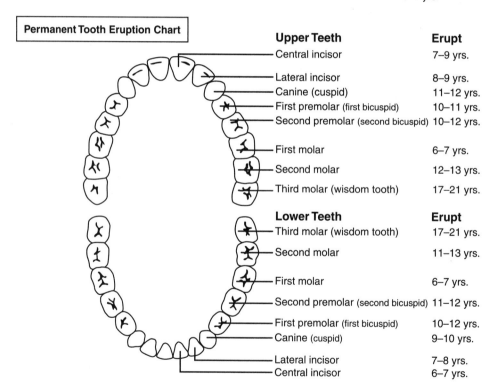

Upper Teeth	Erupt	Shed
Central incisor	8–12 mos.	6–7 yrs.
Lateral incisor	9–13 mos.	7–8 yrs.
Canine (cuspid)	16–22 mos.	10–12 yrs.
First molar	13–19 mos.	9–11 yrs.
Second molar	25–33 mos.	10–12 yrs.

Lower Teeth	Erupt	Shed
Second molar	23–31 mos.	10–12 yrs.
First molar	14–18 mos.	9–11 yrs.
Canine (cuspid)	17–23 mos.	9–12 yrs.
Lateral incisor	10–16 mos.	7–8 yrs.
Central incisor	6–10 mos.	6–7 yrs.

Permanent Tooth Eruption Chart

Upper Teeth	Erupt
Central incisor	7–9 yrs.
Lateral incisor	8–9 yrs.
Canine (cuspid)	11–12 yrs.
First premolar (first bicuspid)	10–11 yrs.
Second premolar (second bicuspid)	10–12 yrs.
First molar	6–7 yrs.
Second molar	12–13 yrs.
Third molar (wisdom tooth)	17–21 yrs.

Lower Teeth	Erupt
Third molar (wisdom tooth)	17–21 yrs.
Second molar	11–13 yrs.
First molar	6–7 yrs.
Second premolar (second bicuspid)	11–12 yrs.
First premolar (first bicuspid)	10–12 yrs.
Canine (cuspid)	9–10 yrs.
Lateral incisor	7–8 yrs.
Central incisor	6–7 yrs.

Source: American Dental Association, *www.ada.org*

Appendix B

Examples of Some Drugs Causing Xerostomia, or Dry Mouth

Brand Name	Generic Name
Anorexiants	
Adiphex-P, Fastin, Ionamin, Zantryl	phentermine
Pondamin, Fen-Phen	fenfluramine
Antiacne	
Accutane	isotretinoin
Antianxiety	
Atarax	hydroxyzine
Ativan	lorazepam
Valium	diazepam
Xanax	alprazolam
Anticholinergic / Antispasmodic	
Atropisol, Sal-Tropine	atropine
Bentyl	dicyclomine
Ditropan	oxybutynin
Transderm-Scop	scopalomine
Anticonvulsant	
Neurontin	Gabapentin
Tegretol	carbamazepine

(*continued*)

Brand Name	Generic Name
Antidepressant	
Elavil	amitriptyline
Prozac	fluoxetine
Sinequan	doxepin
Wellbutrin	buproprine
Antihistamines	
Actifed	triprolidine w/ pseudoephedrine
Benadryl	diphenhydramine
Chlor-trimeton	chlorpheniramine
Claritin	loratadine
Dimetapp	brompheniramine w/ phenylpropanolamine
Seldane	terfenadine
Antihypertensive	
Capoten	captopril
Catepres	clonodine
Minipress	prazosin
Wytensin	guanabenz
Anti-inflammatory Analgesic	
Dolobid	diflunisal
Feldene	piroxicam
Motrin	ibuprofen
Naprosyn	naproxen
Antipsychotic	
Compazine	prochlorperazine
Haldol	haloperidol
Thorazine	chlorpromazine
Bronchodilator	
Atrovent	ipratropium
Isuprel	Isoproterenol
Proventil, Ventolin	Albuterol
Decongestant	
Sudafed	pseudoephedrine

(*continued*)

Brand Name	Generic Name
Diuretic	
Diuril	chlorothiazide
Dyazide, Maxzide	triamterene w/ hydrochlorthiazide
Lasix	flurosemide
Muscle Relaxant	
Flexeril	cyclobenzaprine
Norflex	orphenadrine
Narcotic Analgesic	
Demerol	meperidine
MS Contin	morphine
Sedative	
Halcion	triazolam
Restoril	temazepam

Appendix C

2005 Dietary Guidelines for Americans

Adequate Nutrients Within Calorie Needs

- Consume a variety of nutrient-dense foods and beverages within and among the basic food groups while choosing foods that limit the intake of saturated and trans fats, cholesterol, added sugars, salt, and alcohol.
- Meet recommended intakes within energy needs by adopting a balanced eating pattern, such as the U.S. Department of Agriculture (USDA) Food Guide or the Dietary Approaches to Stop Hypertension (DASH) Eating Plan.

Weight Management

- To maintain body weight in a healthy range, balance calories from foods and beverages with calories expended.
- To prevent gradual weight gain over time, make small decreases in food and beverage calories and increase physical activity.

Physical Activity

- Engage in regular physical activity and reduce sedentary activities to promote health, psychological well-being, and a healthy body weight.
  - To reduce the risk of chronic disease in adulthood: Engage in at least 30 minutes of moderate-intensity physical activity, above usual activity, at work or home on most days of the week.
  - For most people, greater health benefits can be obtained by engaging in physical activity of more vigorous intensity or longer duration.

- To help manage body weight and prevent gradual, unhealthy body weight gain in adulthood: Engage in approximately 60 minutes of moderate- to vigorous-intensity activity on most days of the week while not exceeding caloric intake requirements.
- To sustain weight loss in adulthood: Participate in at least 60 to 90 minutes of daily moderate-intensity physical activity while not exceeding caloric intake requirements. Some people may need to consult with a healthcare provider before participating in this level of activity.
- Achieve physical fitness by including cardiovascular conditioning, stretching exercises for flexibility, and resistance exercises or calisthenics for muscle strength and endurance.

Food Groups To Encourage

- Consume a sufficient amount of fruits and vegetables while staying within energy needs. Two cups of fruit and 2_ cups of vegetables per day are recommended for a reference 2,000-calorie intake, with higher or lower amounts depending on the calorie level.
- Choose a variety of fruits and vegetables each day. In particular, select from all five vegetable subgroups (dark green, orange, legumes, starchy vegetables, and other vegetables) several times a week.
- Consume 3 or more ounce-equivalents of whole-grain products per day, with the rest of the recommended grains coming from enriched or whole-grain products. In general, at least half the grains should come from whole grains.
- Consume 3 cups per day of fat-free or low-fat milk or equivalent milk products.

Fats

- Consume less than 10 percent of calories from saturated fatty acids and less than 300 mg/day of cholesterol, and keep trans fatty acid consumption as low as possible.
- Keep total fat intake between 20 to 35 percent of calories, with most fats coming from sources of polyunsaturated and monounsaturated fatty acids, such as fish, nuts, and vegetable oils.
- When selecting and preparing meat, poultry, dry beans, and milk or milk products, make choices that are lean, low-fat, or fat-free.
- Limit intake of fats and oils high in saturated and/or trans fatty acids, and choose products low in such fats and oils.

Carbohydrates

- Choose fiber-rich fruits, vegetables, and whole grains often.
- Choose and prepare foods and beverages with little added sugars or caloric sweeteners, such as amounts suggested by the USDA Food Guide and the DASH Eating Plan.
- Reduce the incidence of dental caries by practicing good oral hygiene and consuming sugar- and starch-containing foods and beverages less frequently.

Sodium and Potassium

- Consume less than 2,300 mg (approximately 1 teaspoon of salt) of sodium per day.
- Choose and prepare foods with little salt. At the same time, consume potassium-rich foods, such as fruits and vegetables.

Alcoholic Beverages

- Those who choose to drink alcoholic beverages should do so sensibly and in moderation-defined as the consumption of up to one drink per day for women and up to two drinks per day for men.
- Alcoholic beverages should not be consumed by some individuals, including those who cannot restrict their alcohol intake, women of childbearing age who may become pregnant, pregnant and lactating women, children and adolescents, individuals taking medications that can interact with alcohol, and those with specific medical conditions.
- Alcoholic beverages should be avoided by individuals engaging in activities that require attention, skill, or coordination, such as driving or operating machinery.

Food Safety

- To avoid microbial foodborne illness:
  - Clean hands, food contact surfaces, and fruits and vegetables. Meat and poultry should not be washed or rinsed.
  - Separate raw, cooked, and ready-to-eat foods while shopping, preparing, or storing foods.
  - Cook foods to a safe temperature to kill microorganisms.
  - Chill (refrigerate) perishable food promptly and defrost foods properly.
  - Avoid raw (unpasteurized) milk or any products made from unpasteurized milk, raw or partially cooked eggs or foods containing raw eggs, raw or undercooked meat and poultry, unpasteurized juices, and raw sprouts.

Note: The Dietary Guidelines for Americans 2005 contains additional recommendations for specific populations. The full document is available at www.healthierus.gov/dietaryguidelines.

Recommended Daily Allowances

Fat-Soluble Vitamins

Vitamin A	Adult men: 900 g/day	Adult women: 700 g/day
Vitamin D	Adult men & women < age 50:	5 g/day (200 IU)
	Adult men & women age 50–70:	10 g/day (400 IU)
	Adult men & women > age 70:	15 g/day (600 IU)
Vitamin E	Adult men & women:	15 mg-TE
Vitamin K	Adult men: 120 g/day	Adult women: 90 g/day

Water-Soluble Vitamins

Thiamin (Vitamin B1)	Adult men: 1.2 mg	Adult women: 1.1 mg
Riboflavin (Vitamin B2)	Adult men: 1.3 mg	Adult women 1.1 mg
Niacin (Vitamin B3)	Adult men: 16 mg	Adult women: 14 mg
Vitamin B6	Adult men ages 19–50: 1.3 mg >50: 1.7 mg Adult women ages 19–50: 1.3 mg >50: 1.5 mg	
Folate	Adult men and women: 400 g	
Vitamin B12	Adult men and women: 2.4 g	
Vitamin C	Adult men: 90 mg	Adult women: 75 mg

(*Source:* Palmer, Carole A., *Diet and Nutrition in Oral Health*)

Dentition Eruption Tables:

PRIMARY TEETH	Upper Teeth	Erupt	Shed
	Central incisor	8–12 mos.	6–7 yrs.
	Lateral incisor	9–13 mos.	7–8 yrs.
	Canine (cuspid)	16–22 mos.	10–12 yrs.
	First molar	13–19 mos.	9–11 yrs.
	Second molar	25–33 mos.	10–12 yrs.

	Lower Teeth	Erupt	Erupt
	Second molar	23–31 mos.	10–12 yrs.
	First molar	14–18 mos.	9–11 yrs.
	Canine (cuspid)	17–23 mos.	9–12 yrs.
	Lateral incisor	10–16 mos.	7–8 yrs.
	Central incisor	6–10 mos.	6–7 yrs.

(*Source:* Adapted from American Dental Association, www.ada.org)

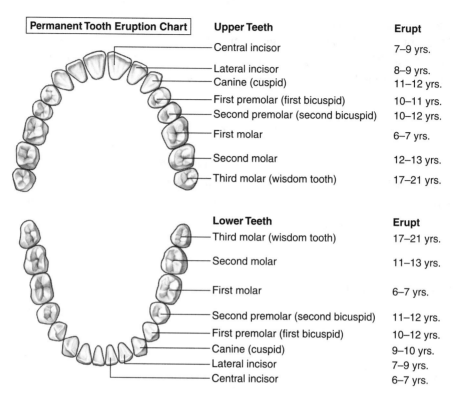

Permanent Tooth Eruption Chart		
Upper Teeth		**Erupt**
Central incisor		7–9 yrs.
Lateral incisor		8–9 yrs.
Canine (cuspid)		11–12 yrs.
First premolar (first bicuspid)		10–11 yrs.
Second premolar (second bicuspid)		10–12 yrs.
First molar		6–7 yrs.
Second molar		12–13 yrs.
Third molar (wisdom tooth)		17–21 yrs.
Lower Teeth		**Erupt**
Third molar (wisdom tooth)		17–21 yrs.
Second molar		11–13 yrs.
First molar		6–7 yrs.
Second premolar (second bicuspid)		11–12 yrs.
First premolar (first bicuspid)		10–12 yrs.
Canine (cuspid)		9–10 yrs.
Lateral incisor		7–9 yrs.
Central incisor		6–7 yrs.

(*Source:* Adapted from American Dental Association, www.ada.org)

Appendix D

Internet Resources

www.adha.org	American Dental Hygienists' Association
www.ada.org	American Dental Association
www.adea.org	American Dental Educators Association
www.ahrq.gov	Agency for Healthcare Research and Quality
www.astdd.org	Association of State and Territorial Dental Directors
www.perio.org	American Academy of Periodontology
www.californiasmokershelpline.org	California Smokers' Helpline
www.cdc.gov	Centers for Disease Control
www.hcfa.gov	Health Care Financing Administration
www.hrsa.gov	U.S. Department of Health and Human Services
www.kansashealth.org	Kansas Health Foundation
www.nidr.nih.gov	National Institute of Dental and Cranofacial Research, National Institute of Health
www.mcn.org	"How to build a team"
www.previser.com	Previser Corporation—*Intercepting Disease*

Note: Internet sites may change. Searching the Internet via key words is another option for obtaining information.

Appendix E

Topics for Basic Oral Health Lessons

1. Toothbrushing
2. Flossing
3. The dental visit: preventive care
4. Tobacco effects/cessation
5. Nutrition: smart food choices/effects of fast foods
6. Plaque control
7. Disease progression: gingivitis/periodontal disease
8. Caring for prostheses: dentures/dental implants
9. Dental care products: toothpastes/rinses
10. Effects of oral piercing
11. Dental safety: mouthguards

Appendix F

Lesson Plan Form

Lesson Plan Form

Target Group: _____   Age Range: _____

Topic for Lesson: _____

Presenter(s): _____

Anticipatory Set (focus):

Purpose (objectives):

Input:

Modeling (show):

Guided Practice (follow me):

Checking for Understanding:

Independent Practice:

Closure:

Appendix G

Plaque Formation Flow Chart/Caries Formation Flow Chart

PLAQUE

Pellicle Formation: an amorphous film forming on the surfaces of teeth, restorations and calculus.
Consists of **glycoproteins**
Influences bacterial colonization

Colonization of Bacteria: bacteria is transported to pellicle via saliva.
Adhere to pellicle
Include - *S. mutans, S. sanguis*
Present: coccal cells

Growth / Maturation: A matrix is formed by bacteria
Present: *S. mutans, S. sanguis, S. mitis, S. salivarius*
Carbohydrates influence adherence to other bacteria and oral surfaces
Actinomyces begins formation
Bacteria continue to grow when undisturbed – decreasing oxygen
Gram+ bacteria decrease
Gram- bacteria increase

Supragingival plaque increases and extends below tissue margin forming subgingival plaque

Crevicular fluid provides nutrients for subgingival plaque

Tissue inflammation begins and increase in severity with increased bacteria and time.

Present: *Porphyromonas, Prevotella, P. intermedia, P. gingivalis, A. actimomycetemcomitans*

CARIES

Development: Microoganisms required (S. mutans) along with a carbohydrate (sucrose), and a susceptible tooth surface

Step I: demineralization from acid products allow bacteria to travel through enamel rods
A white lesion develops

Step II: The white lesion becomes weaker and breaks down forming a soft area on the enamel
The bacteria continue to travel in the direction of the enamel rod (toward pulp)

Step III: The bacteria spreads when contacting the dentinoenamel junction and then follows the direction of the dentinal tubules (toward pulp)

Caries Classification:
Class I   – pits and fissures of occlusal surfaces
Class II – proximal surfaces of premolars / molars
Class III – proximal surfaces of incisors / canines
Class IV – proximal surfaces of incisors / canines
              including the incisal angle
Class V – cervical 1/3 of facial or lingual surfaces
              not including pits or fissures
Class VI – incisal edges of anterior teeth and cusps
              of posterior teeth

Glossary

Active listening—conscious activity based on attitude, attention, and adjustment summarizing what the speaker has said.

Acute necrotizing ulcerative periodontal diseases (ANUP)—a group of destructive, opportunistic gingival/periodontal infections exacerbated by stressors such as tobacco use, nutritional deficiencies, blood dyscrasias, emotional stress, and lack of rest. Bacterial pathogens include spirochetes and Gram-negative organisms that readily invade the tissue, accelerating the destructive nature of these diseases.

Anorexia nervosa—an eating disorder in which the patient has a suppressed or denied appetite. It is more common in young adolescent females and manifests with body weights below normal and obsessive attempts to control or lose weight. Anorexia nervosa is a potentially life-threatening condition.

Bacteremia—microorganisms in the bloodstream.

Biofilm—matrix enclosed bacterial populations adherent to each other and/or surfaces or interfaces.

Body mass index (BMI)—a tool to determine an individual's weight status and possible risk for chronic diseases related to obesity. The formula for BMI is weight/height. BMI of 25–29.9 is considered overweight; above 30 is considered obese.

Bulimia nervosa—an eating disorder in which the patient uses self-induced vomiting and/or laxatives to attempt to compensate for high caloric intakes during binge-eating episodes. The patient with bulimia nervosa is not typically underweight. Oral effects include palatal trauma, enamel erosion, parotid gland enlargement, and xerostomia.

Cariogenicity—a food's potential to contribute to caries occurrence. Example: a food high in fermentable carbohydrates (a soft drink) has a high cariogenicity, whereas a food low in fermentable carbohydrates (a raw carrot) has a low cariogenicity.

Chlorhexidine gluconate—an antiplaque and antigingivitis agent in mouthrinse form.

Chronic obstructive pulmonary disease (COPD)—pulmonary disorders with chronic irreversible obstruction of airflow. Chronic bronchitis and emphysema are the two most common COPDs.

Complimentary proteins—proteins that are incomplete in essential amino acids but when consumed with other incomplete protein foods may result in a complete protein, containing all essential amino acids. Persons choosing to not eat animal proteins must combine incomplete plant proteins in order to meet the body's protein energy needs.

Example: tortillas (lacking lysine) and beans (lacking methionine) are foods with complimentary proteins.

Concrete Operations stage—one of four stages of cognitive development attributed to Jean Piaget, a Swiss psychologist. In this stage, a child (usually between ages 7 and 11) is primarily focused on concrete aspects of their existence while beginning to explore some abstract thought.

Dental anxieties—also referred to as *dental phobias*. Physical and emotional responses to previous negative dental office experiences and/or erroneous impressions of dental care from individuals or media portrayals.

Dental IQ—refers to the dental patient's existing knowledge or awareness of their dental condition, treatment options, and outcomes. This is *not* a reflection of the person's actual intelligence. Assessment of the patient's dental IQ is helpful when developing an individualized oral hygiene education plan.

Early childhood caries (ECC)—rampant caries occurrence in infancy or childhood attributed by improper feeding practices, which allow liquids containing fermentable carbohydrates (breast milk, formula, juices) to pool on the teeth. Carious lesions first appear on the facial surfaces of the upper anterior teeth.

Feedback—a process in which the factors produce a result that are themselves modified, corrected, and strengthened.

Fellow—a graduate student who holds a fellowship in a college or university; a member of a learned society.

Fermentable carbohydrates—monosaccharides, disaccharides, and polysaccharides capable of being used by bacterial plaque as a food source and thus have the potential to lower the plaque pH from neutral to 5.5 or lower.

Fetal alcohol syndrome (FAS)—injury to an unborn baby due to the use of alcohol during pregnancy. FAS may manifest with mental and growth rate retardation, learning and sensory impairments, facial dysmorphologies, and skeletomuscular malformations.

Foundation—an organization established to maintain, assist, or finance institutions, projects, of a social or educational, charitable, or religious, etc., nature.

Fluorosis—a disorder resulting from the absorption of too much fluoride.

Hierarchy of human needs—developed by American psychologist Abraham Maslow as a general guideline for understanding behavior motivations. It may be used by health care providers for insight into individual behaviors and unmet needs.

Infective endocarditis (IE)—a potentially fatal microbial (bacterial, viral, or fungal) infection of the lining of the heart and heart valves. Vegetative growths form on the heart valves, rendering them susceptible to further damage when bacteremia occurs.

Ischemic heart disease—caused by insufficient blood flow from the coronary arteries into the heart and heart tissues.

Neural tube development—early formation of the fetus's spinal cord and nervous system. The neural tube is vulnerable to nutritional effects such as folate deficiencies, resulting in neural tube defects such as spina bifida and anencephaly.

Nidus—a place or substance in an animal or plant where bacteria or other organisms lodge and multiply.

Nutrient-dense foods—foods containing a relatively high level of nutrients, vitamins, and minerals in relation to size or volume. Persons with reduced appetites or eating abilities may be encouraged to consume nutrient-dense foods.

Plaque index—a tool used by dental health care professionals to assess the efficacy of the patient's plaque removal efforts. With modifications, it may be used for group data collection for needs assessments.

PLBW—preterm low birth weight infants. Preventable factors such as cigarette smoking during pregnancy and periodontal disease increase the risk of PLBW infants.

Prophylactic antibiotic premedication—medication administered prior to invasive dental instrumentation to patients at risk of IE.

Prostaglandins—any of a group of hormone-like fatty acids found throughout the body that affects blood pressure, metabolism, body temperature, and other important body processes.

Prothrombin time—a laboratory test used to determine the range of time for blood to clot. Normal range is usually 11–15 seconds; excess of 15 seconds is considered to be prolonged.

Remineralization—replacement of minerals (calcium, phosphate, and fluoride ions) in damaged tooth surfaces; aided by topical fluoride exposures.

Sordes—foul, crusted accumulation forming on the lips, teeth, and oral mucosa of patients with low-grade fevers or not receiving oral hygiene care.

Standard of care—a level of excellence, attainment regarded as a level of adequacy. Generally established in health professions by practitioners.

Target group—a group of individuals selected for a specific goal or objective.

Topical uptake—references benefits of fluoride exposure through surface exposure (fluoridated water, dentifrice, mouthrinse) versus systemic exposure.

24-hour recall—a tool used by health care professionals in the preliminary assessment and determination of the patient's nutritional status and identification of possible excesses or deficiencies. An interview is conducted asking the patient to recall what was consumed during the previous 24 hours, beginning with the most recent meal or snack.

Type II diabetes—non-insulin-dependent diabetes mellitus. Its occurrence is associated with obesity.

Xerostomia—dry mouth caused by medications, salivary gland dysfunctions, radiation therapy of the head or neck regions, or medical conditions such as Sjögren's syndrome. Oral effects include rampant caries, difficulty eating, speaking, or swallowing, and difficulty with denture retention.

Index